MINDFULNESS FOR ADULT ADHD

Mindfulness for Adult ADHD

A CLINICIAN'S GUIDE

Lidia Zylowska
John T. Mitchell

Foreword by Russell A. Barkley

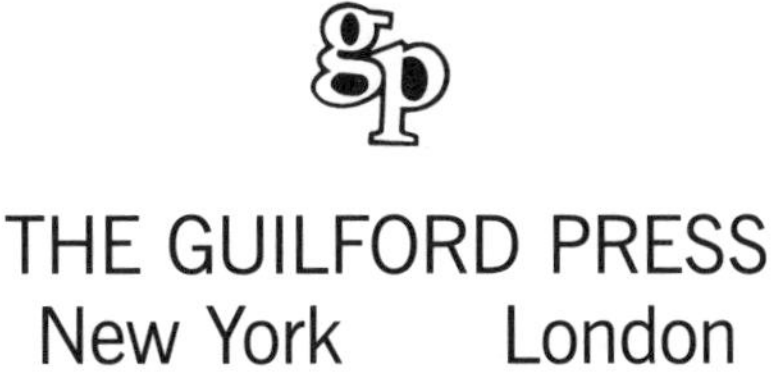

THE GUILFORD PRESS
New York London

A Division of Guilford Publications, Inc.
370 Seventh Avenue, Suite 1200, New York, NY 10001
www.guilford.com

Printed in the United States of America

This book is printed on acid-free paper.

Last digit is print number: 9 8 7 6 5 4 3 2 1

The authors have checked with sources believed to be reliable in their efforts to provide information that is complete and generally in accord with the standards of practice that are accepted at the time of publication. However, in view of the possibility of human error or changes in behavioral, mental health, or medical sciences, neither the authors, nor the editor and publisher, nor any other party who has been involved in the preparation or publication of this work warrants that the information contained herein is in every respect accurate or complete, and they are not responsible for any errors or omissions or the results obtained from the use of such information. Readers are encouraged to confirm the information contained in this book with other sources.

Library of Congress Cataloging-in-Publication Data

Names: Zylowska, Lidia, author. | Mitchell, John T., author.
Title: Mindfulness for adult ADHD : a clinician's guide / Lidia Zylowska, John T. Mitchell ; foreword by Russell A. Barkley
Description: New York : The Guilford Press, [2021] | Includes bibliographical references and index.
Identifiers: LCCN 2020036574 | ISBN 9781462545001 (paperback) | ISBN 9781462544929 (hardcover)
Subjects: LCSH: Attention-deficit disorder in adults—Alternative treatment—Popular works. | Attention-deficit disorder in adults—Alternative treatment—Popular works. | Mind and body therapies—Popular works. | Mind and body therapies—Popular works. | Psychotherapy.
Classification: LCC RC394.A85 Z94 2021 | DDC 616.85/89—dc23
LC record available at *https://lccn.loc.gov/2020036574*

To my husband, Jeff, and my son, Luke:
You are my guides to the richness of the present moment.

—L. Z.

To my wonderful son, Micah,
and my loving parents, Paul and Gerry

—J. T. M.

To everyone living with ADHD
and all the professionals who help them thrive

—L. Z. and J. T. M.

About the Authors

Lidia Zylowska, MD, is Associate Professor in the Department of Psychiatry and Behavioral Sciences at the University of Minnesota and a faculty member at the University's Earl E. Bakken Center for Spirituality and Healing. Dr. Zylowska is a Diplomate of the American Board of Integrative Holistic Medicine. Internationally recognized as an expert in adult attention-deficit/hyperactivity disorder (ADHD) and mindfulness-based therapies, she is a cofounding member of the Mindful Awareness Research Center at the University of California, Los Angeles. Dr. Zylowska pioneered the application of mindfulness in ADHD and led the development of the Mindful Awareness Practices (MAPs) for ADHD Program. She has published articles in peer-reviewed journals and is author of the award-winning self-help book *The Mindfulness Prescription for Adult ADHD.*

John T. Mitchell, PhD, is Assistant Professor in the Department of Psychiatry and Behavioral Sciences at Duke University and a faculty member in Duke's ADHD Program. Dr. Mitchell has published over 65 peer-reviewed journal articles and book chapters, with a primary focus on ADHD, including developmental outcomes, assessment and treatment, and co-occurring substance use. He conducted the first controlled study of a mindfulness-based treatment program—the MAPs for ADHD Program—with a sample composed entirely of adults with ADHD. Dr. Mitchell regularly provides training to clinicians on the assessment and treatment of ADHD in adulthood.

Foreword

If you want to teach mindfulness in your clinical practice with adults with attention-deficit/hyperactivity disorder (ADHD), then this is clearly the best book for achieving this purpose. The authors spell out in exquisite detail not only the compelling rationale for the use of this approach to symptomatic management of adult ADHD, but also the step-by-step instructions for doing so. Included as well are the client handouts to be used in various steps of the program, making this a veritable toolkit for the training of mindfulness practices in ADHD management. Just as informative and useful is the conveyance of the pearls and perils of implementing this approach to treatment—the key issues that contribute to treatment success as well as those that may contribute to not just a poor response but even to potential adverse events or side effects along the way. It is the rare book on mindfulness meditation that even dares to mention what experts in this treatment have long known—effective therapies produce side effects in a significant minority of patients so exposed. It is therefore both a manual of what to do as well as what not to do so as to implement this approach with the hopes of maximal effectiveness. My compliments to the authors for rendering it in so useful a format and with such clinical wisdom.

Interest in applying mindfulness meditation to adults with ADHD actually goes back more than 35 years. I was working as Director of Psychology at the University of Massachusetts Medical Center in Worcester, Massachusetts, and supervising our research clinics for child and adult ADHD when I was approached by a colleague of Dr. Jon Kabat-Zinn wishing to undertake a study of the effectiveness of mindfulness-based stress reduction (MBSR) for adults with ADHD. At the time, Jon and his team, working in the Division of Behavioral Medicine, had developed their MBSR program, as detailed in his book *Full Catastrophe Living,* and were employing it with good success in assisting people with chronic or life-threatening medical illnesses in coping with and reducing the extent of stress and anxiety associated with their conditions. Given the pervasive and serious impairments associated with adult ADHD and especially its core problem with attention, it made sense that someone should study the utility of mindfulness and its focus on attention mechanisms for ADHD in adults. Alas, for various reasons, the study was never initiated. No matter, as Jon's program went on to become exceptionally popular and evidence-based. Indeed it became the most widely adopted program for teaching not only MBSR in clinical settings but mindfulness and its associated meditation in the West, and for coping not only with chronic or life-threatening medical problems but with many other conditions, including the stressors of modern life. And in the past decade, clinical researchers such as the authors of this book have returned to study the effectiveness of MBSR for adults with ADHD in more detail and with greater rigor than initial attempts had done.

As the authors rightly note in their own rationale for undertaking to lay out the details of this approach, adult ADHD is far more than just a disorder of attention. It is a disorder of executive functioning (EF) and self-regulation. And among the various components that MBSR might be able to address are not just its problems with attentional focus and persistence of such but emotional impulsivity and poor emotional self-regulation. Thus, it makes good sense to further explore the utility of mindfulness for ADHD in adults and especially these EF deficits, among others.

We now have a larger body of evidence and some very carefully designed research efforts showing that mindfulness training of adults with ADHD has great promise even though it may be less efficacious for children with the disorder. Despite my earlier skepticism, findings reported in several meta-analyses of the growing body of research on mindfulness training for adult ADHD have led me to view this treatment as a highly promising, albeit still experimental, approach. There is clearly a treatment effect of some sort associated with this approach to ADHD management, especially in comparison to no treatment, wait-list control groups. As the authors rightly note in Chapter 2, the few studies that have compared mindful awareness practices (MAPs) or other mindfulness training methods for ADHD to other active interventions or information/attention control groups find that both approaches improve outcome measures but may not differ in their results. In that sense, mindfulness may be as good as information-based therapies for ADHD or alternative cognitive-behavioral interventions—and for some outcome measures, maybe better. This manual offers the prospect of promoting efforts by others to conduct further well-controlled studies of mindfulness training by its provision of a standardized approach that is spelled out in detail and that can be implemented in a variety of clinical settings and, importantly, with some possibility of fidelity to the original MAPs methods. Let us hope that it does so, as we can use many more evidence-based psychosocial approaches to adult ADHD besides the medications often used in its management.

In the meantime, I congratulate the authors for setting forth here so detailed a clinical manual as to make it relatively easy and straightforward to implement the MAPs approach to ADHD management in a convenient, easily understood, and now widely available format. This manual expands the previously limited array of clinically available psychosocial (nonmedical) approaches to the management of ADHD in adults. And it offers those adults an alternative form of therapy that, according to recent research, is rated by clients as among the most useful components of any package of ADHD interventions they have been offered.

RUSSELL A. BARKLEY, PhD
Virginia Commonwealth University Medical Center

Preface

"So you plan to have people who have trouble sitting still and paying attention to sit and pay attention in meditation? Isn't this a set-up for failure and frustration?" This was a question posed to one of us (Lidia Zylowska) many years ago when she was first designing a research program in mindfulness and attention-deficit/hyperactivity disorder (ADHD). The question was fair, yet missing the perspective that mindfulness meditation can be a remediation strategy for ADHD. By remediation, we mean identifying where the weakness is in ADHD and through practice strengthening the skill. So if sitting still and paying attention is a weakness in ADHD, why not strengthen the weakness via mental exercises of mindfulness practice the way physical exercise can strengthen a weak leg? After all, meditation is at its heart a training of attention and learning to regulate emotions and impulses, including restlessness. As more research in this area evolved, this perspective and its rationale have also evolved, highlighting that ADHD is a self-awareness and self-regulation disorder and mindfulness practice—sitting meditation *and* other informal ways such as mindfulness in daily life, mindful movement, and compassion practice—are self-awareness and self-regulation training.

Following this premise that mindfulness can strengthen the ADHD-related deficits of self-regulation, Lidia started the initial mindfulness for ADHD research in 2003 at UCLA. Supported by a Robert Wood Johnson Fellowship, in collaboration with ADHD researcher Sue Smalley, PhD, she led the first pilot study of mindfulness-based intervention with adults and teens with ADHD. This initial study created the Mindful Awareness Practices—or MAPs—for ADHD Program, which was designed to be ADHD-friendly by including ADHD education and modifying mindfulness practice to be gradual and versatile. The promising results of this initial pilot ignited tremendous interest in mindfulness-based interventions for ADHD. The program also helped establish the UCLA Mindful Awareness Research Center and its other MAPs training. Soon after (in 2009), Lidia met John Mitchell, PhD (this book's coauthor), from Duke University. John was preparing to conduct the first pilot randomized controlled trial using the MAPs for ADHD Program for adults with ADHD after receiving funding from the American Professional Society of ADHD and Related Disorders and The Pond

Family Foundation. We began a dialogue about our shared interest in mindfulness for ADHD. Over the years, we have had a continued dialogue on using MAPs in clinical and research settings. We worked together on articles reviewing the scientific rationale and evidence for mindfulness in ADHD, as well as potential adverse effects. We both have been active in supporting other researchers and clinicians interested in this approach by sharing our experience via collaborations or presentations. We have been excited to see a growth in number of studies validating the value of mindfulness-based interventions for ADHD, especially adult ADHD. However, as we went along, we realized a need for an up-to-date clinical manual that researchers and providers could use in their work with adults with ADHD. This clinician's guide was written to meet this need and to make this approach more available to patients.

This book is divided into three separate parts: (1) a section that provides an overview and conceptual foundation for the administration of the MAPs for ADHD Program; (2) a session-by-session MAPs for ADHD treatment manual; and (3) a section that addresses considerations once an adult with ADHD completes this treatment. We attempted to be consistent in our use of language and abbreviations. As we describe in Chapter 1, we adopt the term "mindfulness trainer" (MT) as an inclusive term to refer to any instructor (e.g., psychologist, psychotherapist, physician, ADHD coach) who may be providing this treatment. We also attempted to be consistent in our use of "MAPs" to refer specifically to the Mindfulness Awareness Practices for ADHD Program. Our use of boldface was also purposeful throughout the book to emphasize concepts or themes, as well as to provide a structure for subsections within each chapter.

Part II is the session-by-session treatment manual that provides guidance on how to administer MAPs. While we want readers to approach MAPs with a strong understanding of its framework and grasp the practical aspects of its administration, our overarching intention is for MTs to consider MAPs as an adaptable treatment to meet the needs of the adults with ADHD they work with. Therefore, we hope that this book inspires MTs to use their own creativity and build on the foundation and structure that MAPs provides. We attempt to model this adaptability by providing recommendations on how to modify MAPs for an individual therapy setting. We do this because, while MAPs was developed and tested in a group therapy format much like other mindfulness-based interventions from which it was derived, there may be circumstances in which adapting the approach for individual therapy is warranted.

Then, in Part III we provide guidance on future directions to consider as the initial 8-week MAPs training is concluding. Treatment options post-MAPs may take many different forms depending on the clinical context. We attempt to provide treatment considerations that will be applicable for most adults with ADHD.

One part of MAPs is weekly, at-home guided meditations. These guided meditations referred to in the session-by-session portion of this book can be found in the book *The Mindfulness Prescription for Adult ADHD* (Zylowska, 2012) or on The Guilford Press website (see the box at the end of the table of contents). Since *The Mindfulness Prescription for Adult ADHD* can be thought of as an early self-help version of this manual, the MT may find it helpful to recommend this resource to adults with ADHD who are participating in MAPs.

Finally, our overarching hope is that this manual will lead to further research and clinical refinement of mindfulness-based interventions in ADHD and help establish the use of this approach in ADHD across the lifespan.

Acknowledgments

This book reflects our mutual interest and work in mindfulness for attention-deficit/hyperactivity disorder (ADHD). We met in 2012 after Lidia published her Mindful Awareness Practices (MAPs) for ADHD Program study funded by the Robert Wood Johnson Foundation and wrote her first book, *The Mindfulness Prescription for Adult ADHD.* At that time, John received a grant from the American Professional Society of ADHD and Related Disorders and The Pond Family Foundation to further study mindfulness in ADHD. This initial meeting has led to a rewarding collaboration over the years, and we are both grateful for the opportunity to now share with you our joint experience via this book.

Many people have been instrumental in supporting our work in mindfulness for ADHD and without them, this treatment and this book would not be what it is now. We want to acknowledge all the important work done by the original teachers of mindfulness-based stress reduction (Jon Kabat-Zinn and Saki Santorelli) and mindfulness-based cognitive therapy (Mark G. Williams, John D. Teasdale, and Zindel Segal) that formed a foundation for the MAPs for ADHD Program. We are also indebted to our colleagues at the University of California, Los Angeles (Lidia) and Duke University (John) who supported our initial work in this area, particularly Susan Smalley, Kenneth Wells, and Scott Kollins. Their support was instrumental as it was years before the utility of mindfulness for ADHD was widely recognized. John would also like to thank his graduate school advisor, Rosemery Nelson-Gray, who helped lay a foundation that emphasized the importance of a scientific and compassionate approach to clinical care. We want to thank the countless patients, students, clinicians, scientists, and the ADHD community who have shown interest in this approach over the years and shared their own insights in engaging with mindfulness. In making this book, we especially want to thank Lee Freedman for insightful conversations about mindfulness and ADHD; Kathleen Nadeau and Russ Ramsay for an early read of this book; and Russell A. Barkley for his foreword. We also want to thank Senior Editor Jim Nageotte, who believed in this book even when the early manuscript was at a publishing crossroads, and the Guilford team for bringing this book to publication. Last, but not least, we want to thank our families for their love and support during the many months of writing this book.

Contents

Purchasers of this book can download and print enlarged versions of the reproducible session summaries and handouts as well as access recorded guided meditations at *www.guilford.com/zylowska-materials* for personal use or use with clients (see copyright page for details).

PART I

OVERVIEW

Knowing the "Why" before the "What"

The first four chapters of this book provide a foundation in practical, conceptual, and empirical issues involving mindfulness for attention-deficit/hyperactivity disorder (ADHD). This includes a brief introduction to orient readers (Chapter 1), a conceptual and research review on the use of mindfulness-based interventions for ADHD in adulthood (Chapter 2), common questions and answers that arise when learning the Mindful Awareness Practices (MAPs) for ADHD Program (Chapter 3), and ADHD psychoeducation topics that are taught in MAPs (Chapter 4).

CHAPTER 1

Introduction

Welcome!

We are glad to see your interest in mindfulness training for adults with attention-deficit/hyperactivity disorder (ADHD). We believe that mindfulness training offers strategies that are new to and needed in the field of ADHD. In this chapter, we provide a brief introduction to mindfulness, discuss the benefits of mindfulness training for ADHD, outline the Mindful Awareness Practices (MAPs) for ADHD Program (which we discuss in detail in Part II of the book), and provide a general orientation to this manual.

Mindfulness (or as we often call it, mindful awareness) is *a practice of being attentive to and accepting of experiences in the present moment*. This mental practice is typically done in silent meditation, but can also be trained in the course of daily activities. By repeatedly engaging in instances of monitoring one's experience, the practice encourages moving attention away from busy mental activity or self-narrative focus to moment-by-moment noting of sensory input (e.g., sounds or breath sensations) and meta-awareness of emotional, cognitive, and sensory reactions. Overall, mindfulness is recognized as a multifaceted approach that develops attention and emotional *self-regulation*, and offers new choices in responding. Through new mindfulness skills, patients can engage in their day-to-day experience in a different, more adaptive way.

ADHD is a self-regulation disorder; mindfulness is self-regulation training.

BENEFITS OF MINDFULNESS TRAINING IN ADHD

While mindfulness for ADHD research is still evolving (see Chapter 2 for a detailed review of recent studies), current evidence and conceptual understanding of both mindfulness and ADHD suggest the following benefits in ADHD:

- *Attention self-regulation.* Training of attention stability and flexibility, and improved control over mind wandering. While the first letters in the ADHD acronym indicate an attention deficit, ADHD is more akin to an attention regulation disorder. Relatedly, mindfulness strengthens executive functioning and protects working memory from depletion when under stress—the very cognitive resources involved in regulation of attention.
- *Emotional self-regulation.* Improved emotional awareness, reappraisal of negative emotions, willingness to experience and be affected by previously avoided emotions, and decreased inner reactivity and emotional impulsivity (i.e., acting impulsively in the context of strong emotions).
- *New response choices and new adaptive behaviors.* For example, increased nonjudgmental awareness of distractibility can invite more frequent self-directed correction of attention. This creates new opportunities to notice the effectiveness of single-tasking (as opposed to multitasking) and greater likelihood of completing a task.
- *Change in the perspective on the self.* Detachment from a fixed sense of self as self-understanding increases through expanded knowledge of one's brain function, ADHD patterns, and internal resources to deal with challenges.
- *Self-compassion.* Developing a more supportive, compassionate relationship with oneself, which counteracts shame, stigma, and self-judgments frequently found in ADHD; overall improved self-acceptance.
- *Improvement in stress management and mental resilience skills.*
- *Improvement in interpersonal communication.*

THE MAPs FOR ADHD APPROACH

MAPs for ADHD was originally developed at UCLA in the course of a feasibility study by Lidia Zylowska and Susan Smalley (Zylowska et al., 2008). This group-based training is modeled after mindfulness-based stress reduction (MBSR; Kabat-Zinn, 1990) and mindfulness-based cognitive therapy (MBCT; Segal et al., 2002), with adaptations made for individuals diagnosed with ADHD. Other influences include the Vipassana meditation tradition, acceptance-based therapies, and ADHD psychosocial approaches.

Meditation—a practice typically associated with sitting still and paying attention—can be difficult and discouraging to those with a condition like ADHD that is characterized by frequent restlessness and wandering focus. Thus, the intention behind designing this program was to make it gradual and overall ADHD-friendly. The following adaptations were included:

1. Psychoeducation on the clinical symptoms, neurobiology, and etiology of ADHD is woven throughout the training.
2. Training is step-wise, with sessions 1–3 emphasizing control of attention and

moving away from "automatic pilot mode" such as distracted or busy mind, and sessions 4–8 applying meta-awareness skills to inner experiences.

3. Formal meditation periods are shorter than in other similar programs (e.g., in an MBSR program, 45 minutes of at-home practice is recommended, and in MAPs for ADHD, formal practice is 5- to 15-minutes long).
4. Didactic visual aids are included to address different learning styles.
5. Strategies from ADHD cognitive-behavioral therapy and coaching are used to facilitate mindful awareness practice.
6. At the end of each session, an appreciation meditation or loving-kindness meditation (an exercise of wishing-well to self and others) is included to address the low self-esteem frequently found in ADHD.

To balance intensity of the training and allow for ease of delivery within diverse clinical and research settings, the MAPs for ADHD Program does not include a half-day retreat typically included in MBSR or MBCT. Similarly, while body awareness is practiced throughout the training in several ways (e.g., walking, short movement and stretching exercises, body-breath-sound meditation, and mindfulness of emotions), longer (45 minutes) body scan and yoga poses typically used in MBSR and MBCT are not included. Overall, the MAPs for ADHD Program is designed as a beginning instruction in mindful awareness suitable for individuals who may otherwise not easily engage with meditation practice, including beginners or those with mental health challenges (of note, the MAPs for ADHD Program has provided the basis for another similar introductory course, MAPS I, that is now offered at the UCLA Mindful Awareness Research Center for the general population).

The MAPs for ADHD Program was initially designed for groups of older adolescents (15–18 years old) and adults with ADHD. Originally described in 2008 (Zylowska et al., 2008, 2009), the training was further expanded in a self-help book (Zylowska, 2012), which can support adaptation for individual therapy as well. Since the MAPs for ADHD Program has been researched as a group intervention with ADHD adults with promising empirical support, this manual focuses on a group format for ADHD adults. For clinicians wishing to use it in individual therapy cases and/or with younger ages, within each session we include tips based on our and other clinicians' experience with such delivery.

It is important to note that mindfulness is both a natural capacity and a skill strengthened by mental practice. Our approach assumes that both formal mindfulness (i.e., silent periods of sitting or walking meditation) and informal mindfulness (i.e., brief "mindful check-ins" throughout daily activities) can strengthen the natural capacity and benefit those with ADHD. Although research evidence is yet to tease out what practice provides what benefits, our approach is that patients should be given diverse options of how to train in mindfulness. We want to empower those with ADHD to find their own way of practicing and keeping mindfulness in their lives. Formal and informal practice is seen as equally beneficial and encouraged throughout the training.

HOW IS THIS BOOK ORGANIZED?

The book has three main parts:

- Part I: Introduction, review of mindfulness for ADHD research, and overview of framework for using a mindfulness-based approach in ADHD (see Chapters 1–4).
- Part II: Session-by-session detailed description of the MAPs for ADHD Program. Teaching scripts are included to help group facilitators with the training delivery. The sessions are designed for training in a group therapy setting, but we also include tips on how to adapt this teaching to individual therapy sessions (see Sessions 1–8).
- Part III: Considerations for what to do after the initial MAPs for ADHD training is completed.

This book also contains an Appendix with patient handouts and session outlines for clinicians to share with group members at the clinician's discretion.

WHO COULD BENEFIT FROM USING THIS BOOK?

This book is primarily for clinicians or other mental health professionals working with adults with ADHD. Professionals who could use this approach include psychologists, psychiatrists, other psychotherapy professionals, ADHD coaches, learning disabilities (LD) specialists, and college counselors. Mindfulness or yoga professional teachers can also find this manual helpful, especially if they engage in delivering mind-body training in schools, clinical, or work settings. Those working with children or teens with ADHD can also use and/or modify strategies included in this book—indeed, as you'll see in Chapter 2, some research has already been done extending the MAPs for ADHD approach developmentally "downward" for adolescents. One assumption this manual makes is that the clinician or trainer—throughout this book, we adopt the term "mindfulness trainer," or MT—has a good working knowledge of ADHD as a disorder and its manifestation in adults. For those less familiar with ADHD in adulthood, we recommend gaining further familiarity of the scientific literature, which has been thoroughly summarized in a variety of comprehensive books (see Barkley, 2015; Barkley, Murphy, & Fischer, 2008; Hinshaw & Ellison, 2015; Nigg, 2006).

Since the MAPs for ADHD approach is for adults with ADHD, any patients or clients receiving this treatment—we use the term "participants" throughout the remainder of the book—are assumed to have received a comprehensive diagnostic assessment for ADHD following DSM-5 or ICD-10 criteria. In Chapter 4, we review the current DSM-5 criteria and other common characteristics associated with adult ADHD. For additional, in-depth guidance on the diagnostic process, we refer readers to other books devoted to this topic (see Goldstein & Teeter Ellison, 2002; Kooj, 2013), as well as comprehensive clinical workbooks (see Barkley & Murphy, 2006).

HOW CAN MINDFULNESS BE INCORPORATED INTO ADHD CARE?

Mindfulness-based approaches can complement other commonly used treatments such as medications, cognitive-behavioral therapy, or coaching. Indeed, as you'll see in Chapter 2, mindfulness-based interventions like the MAPs for ADHD Program are considered part of the same family of therapy as cognitive-behavioral therapy. However, by developing self-regulation skills via novel strategies, mindfulness may reduce the need for other treatments or it can optimize well-being while other treatments like medications or psychotherapy are continued. In other words, whether mindfulness is an alternative or complementary training to other treatments, it can improve the daily lives of adults diagnosed with ADHD.

CHAPTER 2

Conceptual and Research Review

Mindfulness-based interventions (MBIs) emerged in the late 1970s with the work of Dr. Jon Kabat-Zinn when he developed MBSR. This intervention utilized silent meditation and yoga practice as key components of treatment. MBSR was initially applied to adults with chronic pain and provided a complementary approach to traditional pain management practices (Kabat-Zinn, 1982; Kabat-Zinn, Lipworth, & Burney, 1985). Additional treatments began to emerge that also used meditation and other mindfulness strategies as the core treatment approach, most notably MBCT for adults with major depressive disorder (Segal et al., 2002). In parallel with the development and refinement of these MBIs into the 1980s and 1990s, a broader class of interventions now referred to as the "third generation" or "third wave" of behavior therapy emerged. This class of interventions had an emphasis on acceptance and mindfulness strategies that could be used in the course of behavior change (Hayes, Follette, & Linehan, 2004; Hayes, Luoma, Bond, Masuda, & Lillis, 2006). Such therapies include acceptance and commitment therapy (ACT; Hayes, Strosahl, & Wilson, 1999, 2012) and dialectical behavior therapy (DBT; Linehan, 1993). These other third-wave therapies incorporate mindfulness practices but teach other nonmindfulness techniques as well. Because of these differences, MBIs such as MBSR and MBCT are considered part of this third wave, but not all third-wave therapies are considered MBIs.

WHAT IS MINDFULNESS?

MBIs have garnered increasing scientific interest only in the past 15 years or so; however, they are derived from a long-standing Eastern tradition of meditation called *Vipassana,* which means "seeing things as they really are." MBIs teach mindfulness via formal meditation practice and informal practices, though the field has yet to define the construct of *mindfulness* in a way that fully addresses the complex, multifaceted Buddhist phenomenology from which it is derived (Bodhi, 2011; Dreyfus, 2011; Dunne, 2011; Gethin, 2011; Grossman, 2008, 2011; Kang & Whittingham, 2010). The term *mindfulness* itself is translated from the Pali word *sati* and has also been translated as including "attention," "awareness," "retention or remembering," and "discernment" (Davidson & Kaszniak, 2015). In the scientific literature, one widely used definition is that mindfulness involves adopting a nonjudgmental attention to one's experience(s) in the present moment (Kabat-Zinn, 1990). Others have defined it as a psychological process comprised of two components: orienting one's attention purposefully to the present moment and approaching one's experience in the present moment with curiosity, openness, and acceptance (Bishop et al., 2004). Another commonly cited definition conceptualizes mindfulness as a trait or set of skills, such as being nonreactive, observing with awareness, acting with awareness, describing with awareness, and adopting a nonjudgmental approach toward one's experience (Baer et al., 2008).

Treatments like MBSR teach two different types of meditation practices: focused monitoring and open monitoring (Lutz, Slagter, Dunne, & Davidson, 2008). MBIs typically begin with an emphasis on focused attention exercises, which involve directing and maintaining a focused attention on something particular, such as the sensation of breathing. When distraction or mind wandering occurs, patients are taught to identify the loss of focus without judgment and reestablish attention toward the original object of focus. As most MBIs progress and focused-monitoring techniques are established, open-monitoring techniques are introduced. With open monitoring, there is no explicit object or sensation to focus on. Instead, patients are taught to be alert, open, and receptive to whatever arises in their awareness in a calm and welcoming manner. Experiences that arise are allowed to essentially come and go on their own accord. When these experiences do arise, patients are taught to be fully present and in the moment with whatever they are. The calm and unattached observation during focused- or open-monitoring practices allows for greater insight into one's own behavior and provides a foundation for more intentional and purposeful behavior. For additional discussion of different meditation practices, see Chiesa and Malinowski (2011).

MBIs teach two different types of formal practices: (1) focused monitoring and (2) open monitoring.

MBIs FOR DIVERSE PSYCHIATRIC AND MEDICAL GROUPS

Current State of Research Evidence

For readers wanting to learn more about the state of research on MBIs, this box provides a general overview of MBI treatment literature across populations other than ADHD. For additional in-depth discussions see special issues of peer-reviewed journals devoted to MBIs (e.g., Baer, 2016; Black, 2014; Davidson & Kaszniak, 2015; DeSole, 2011; Renshaw & Cook, 2017; Tang & Posner, 2013).

Across MBI treatment studies, nearly half, 45%, are Stage I trials (Dimidjian & Segal, 2015). These studies involve intervention creation, modification, adaptation, or refinement (Stage IA) and feasibility and pilot testing (Stage IB). Stage II efficacy trials make up about 29% of these studies: 20% are trials that include a wait-list control condition or a treatment-as-usual condition, and 9% are trials that include an active-treatment control condition. With an additional 25% of MBI treatment studies at the Stage 0 level that are at a more basic level of research examining intervention targets and mechanisms of change, fewer than 3% of trials have been dedicated to Stages III–V that involve efficacy in the community and broader implementation and dissemination (Dimidjian & Segal, 2015). This type of research progression for an intervention is promising and indicative of the incremental process in treatment development.

There are multiple reviews examining the impact of MBIs for a variety of medical conditions, including chronic pain, diabetes, irritable bowel syndrome, asthma, and insomnia (Chiesa & Serretti, 2011a; Crowe et al., 2016; Loucks et al., 2015; Mikolasek, Berg, Witt, & Barth, 2018; Noordali, Cumming, & Thompson, 2017). In a meta-analysis of 553 adult patients from six different randomized controlled trials (RCTs) recruited from a primary care setting with a variety of conditions (e.g., chronic musculoskeletal pain, chronic illness), the overall effect size on improving general health favoring MBI in comparison to a control condition was moderate (Demarzo et al., 2015). Beneficial effects were also reported for mental health variables and quality of life. In another meta-analysis of a variety of medical samples (n = 8,683) in 115 RCTs, MBIs significantly improved depressive symptoms, anxiety symptoms, stress, quality of life, and physical functioning (Gotink et al., 2015). Meta-analyses and reviews of patients with particular medical diagnoses similarly yield promising results supporting the effects of MBIs. For example, MBIs yield moderate to large effect sizes when assessing stress, depressed mood, anxiety, and state mindfulness in cancer patients (Piet, Wurtzen, & Zachariae, 2012; Zainal, Booth, & Huppert, 2013). Increasingly, mindfulness is also studied in medical practitioners showing that physicians report less burnout after MBI interventions, indirectly benefiting patient care (Krasner et al., 2009).

MBIs have also been actively studied in psychiatric samples as well. In one meta-analysis of 209 studies across different psychiatric and medical groups (n = 12,145 patients), MBIs outperformed wait-list control groups with moderate effect sizes that were maintained at follow-up assessments (Khoury et al., 2013). In comparison to active-treatment groups, MBIs also had a significant effect, but did not differ from empirically supported behavioral or pharmacological treatments. Similarly, in other meta-analyses of MBIs across a range of conditions including psychiatric groups, MBIs have a moderate effect for improving anxiety and depressive symptoms. Of note, large effect sizes emerge when analyses are restricted to patients with anxiety and mood disorders (Hofmann, Sawyer, Witt, & Oh, 2010). Additional reviews indicate support for MBIs (e.g., Chen et al., 2012; Chiesa & Serretti, 2011b; Fjorback, Arendt, Ornbol, Fink, & Walach, 2011; Galante, Iribarren, & Pearce, 2013). In one meta-analysis of RCTs in adult patients with recurrent major depressive episodes (n = 1,258), MBCT was associated with reduced risk of depressive episode relapse within a 60-week follow-up period in comparison to those who had treatment as usual (Kuyken et al., 2016). Interestingly, these results were not restricted to particular sociodemographic variables, including age, sex, education, and relationship status.

MBIs have also been actively examined in substance use samples. For instance, in a meta-analysis of four RCTs including 474 adult cigarette smokers, 25.2% of those who received mindfulness training were abstinent from smoking for more than 4 months versus 13.6% of those who received standard smoking cessation treatment (Oikonomou, Arvanitis, & Sokolove, 2017). Other reviews indicate that MBIs improve various other forms of substance abuse (e.g., alcohol, cocaine, amphetamines) and may reduce drug craving as well (Chiesa & Serretti, 2014; Zgierska et al., 2009). In a trial examining relapse prevention among substance-abusing patients who recently completed intensive outpatient or inpatient care, participants were randomized to a MBI, a cognitive behavioral relapse-prevention training program, or treatment as usual (i.e., 12-step program and psychoeducation). While the first two treatments were superior at posttreatment in terms of reduced relapse risk to drug use and heavy drinking, at 12-month follow-up MBI outperformed the other two treatments for both drug use and heavy drinking (Bowen et al., 2014).

RATIONALE FOR USING MBIs FOR ADHD

MBIs are efficacious for a variety of conditions—both physical and psychiatric disorders. One potential reason for the impact of MBIs in so many different disorders is that MBIs are thought to impact transdiagnostic processes that improve self-regulation. Since ADHD is conceptualized as a self-regulation disorder, applying MBIs to ADHD appears especially fitting. Indeed, in multiple reviews on the topic of MBIs, ADHD has been identified as a particularly compelling disorder with which to assess the effects of mindfulness training given the proposed mechanisms of action of this intervention on attentional processes and related cognitive control capabilities (Chiesa, Calati, & Serretti, 2011; Hölzel et al., 2011; Keng, Smoski, & Robins, 2011).

Impact on Cognitive Processes

Attention Regulation and Executive Functions

Poor attentional functioning is a core symptom cluster of ADHD (American Psychiatric Association, 2013) and associated executive-functioning deficits in ADHD are common (Barkley, 1997; Boonstra, Oosterlaan, Sergeant, & Buitelaar, 2005; Hervey, Epstein, & Curry, 2004). Treatments that appear to improve these processes would indicate that they may improve ADHD outcomes. As we have previously reviewed (Mitchell, Zylowska, & Kollins, 2015), in non-ADHD samples MBIs improve cognitive processes, including attention regulation and executive functioning. At the clinical level, initial mindfulness practices teach patients to focus attention on a particular object (e.g., one's own breath) and to return to this object after becoming distracted. This is proposed to improve attentional control abilities (Keng et al., 2011). More specifically, this practice requires top-down regulation of attention and conflict detection, which can be thought of as a regulatory approach to attention that improves executive processes (Chiesa et al., 2011). Consistent with this proposal, studies examining the effects of meditation practices, even short duration practice, demonstrate improvements. For instance, one study assessed the impact of 5 days (20 minutes per day) of meditation against relaxation (Tang et al., 2007). Posttreatment, the meditation group performed significantly better on conflict detection during an attentional task than the relaxation group. Similar findings have been reported following 4 days of meditation training (20 minutes per day) on visuospatial processing, working memory, and executive functioning against an active-treatment comparison group (Zeidan, Johnson, Diamond, David, & Goolkasian, 2010). Such findings are consistent with neuroimaging studies that support that mindfulness meditation practices result in neuroplastic changes in areas associated with attentional and executive processes. For instance, Hölzel and colleagues (2011) discuss the impact of mindfulness practice on the anterior cingulate cortex, which is involved with executive/attentional processes via detection of conflicting or incompatible incoming information. Suboptimal activation of this area has been identified in ADHD samples (e.g., Cubillo, Halari, Smith, Taylor, & Rubia, 2012; Passarotti, Sweeney, & Pavuluri, 2010). For more on this topic, see Bachmann and colleagues' excellent review of cognitive processes and related brain mechanisms implicated in the use of MBIs for ADHD (Bachmann, Lam, & Philipsen, 2016).

Mind Wandering and Default Mode Network

The phenomenon of mind wandering has many similarities with models of cognitive control (Smallwood & Schooler, 2006). Mind wandering is associated with neural networks of the brain involved with self-referential processing, also known as the default mode network (Christoff, Gordon, Smallwood, Smith, & Schooler, 2009; Mason et al., 2007; Raichle et al., 2001). The networks that make up the default mode network are typically suppressed during attention tasks. This network is not deactivated as well in ADHD as it is in non-ADHD peers (Fair et al., 2010) and is associated with poorer attention regulation in ADHD (Castellanos et al., 2008), including mind wandering (Sonuga-Barke & Castellanos, 2007). See Mowlem and colleagues (2019) for examples of how mind wandering manifests in ADHD.

We and others have previously proposed that impact on the default mode network and associated mind wandering may be another mechanism of action that makes MBIs particularly applicable to ADHD (Bachmann et al., 2016; Mitchell et al., 2015). For example, pharmacological interventions that improve ADHD symptoms normalize activity within this network (Liddle et al., 2011; Peterson et al., 2009). Although studies have not been conducted examining the effects of MBI practices in an ADHD sample on the default mode network and associated mind wandering, studies in non-ADHD samples are promising. For example, there are gray matter differences in the default mode network in long-term meditators (Kurth, MacKenzie-Graham, Toga, & Luders, 2015). In another study, central areas of the default mode network (i.e., medial prefrontal and posterior cortices) were deactivated across different types of meditation exercises among experienced meditators relative to meditation-naïve participants (Brewer et al., 2011). Further, this study indicated stronger functional connectivity between regions involved in self-monitoring and cognitive control (i.e., the posterior cingulate, dorsal anterior cingulate, and dorsolateral prefrontal cortices). Similar differential connectivity between default mode network regions (i.e., dorsomedial prefrontal cortex and right inferior parietal lobule) have emerged in other studies comparing experienced and beginner meditators during a restful state brain scan (Taylor et al., 2013). These findings are consistent with other studies of experienced meditators and associated markers of mind wandering (Ellamil et al., 2016; Hasenkamp, Wilson-Mendenhall, Duncan, & Barsalou, 2012). Although these studies were in experienced meditators, findings indicate generalizability in meditation novices. For example, Brewer and Garrison review how improvement in the default mode network can be taught in meditation novices using real-time functional magnetic resonance imaging (fMRI) feedback (Brewer & Garrison, 2014). Mrazek and colleagues have also demonstrated that MBI training can improve mind wandering in the laboratory (Mrazek, Franklin, Phillips, Baird, & Schooler, 2013; Mrazek, Smallwood, & Schooler, 2012).

Impact on Emotion Dysregulation

Although poor emotion regulation is not a diagnostic feature of ADHD, it is a characteristic of the disorder and some have argued it is a core feature of the disorder (Barkley, 2010). Clinical manifestations of disrupted emotional regulation process in ADHD include impatience, quickness to anger/get upset, being easily frustrated, emotional overreacting, and being easily excited (Barkley, 2010). Such difficulties in emotion regulation often contribute to significant impairment (Barkley & Fischer, 2010; Barkley & Murphy, 2010; Mitchell, Robertson, Anastopolous, Nelson-Gray, & Kollins, 2012).

Though there is no consistently agreed upon definition of "emotion dysregulation," most accounts describe it as a multidimensional construct. As an alternative to emotional intensity or reactivity, one widely accepted definition emphasizes the functionality of emotions and involves (1) a lack of awareness, understanding, and acceptance of emotions; (2) a lack of access to adaptive strategies for modulating the intensity and/or duration of emotional responses; (3) an unwillingness to experience emotional distress as part of pursuing desired goals; and (4) the inability to engage in goal-directed behaviors when experiencing distress (Gratz & Roemer, 2004; Mennin, Heimberg, Turk, & Fresco, 2005). This definition is similar to those adopted in the ADHD literature. For example, Shaw and colleagues define it as the ability to modify an emotion state in the service of adaptive and goal-oriented behavior (Shaw, Stringaris, Nigg, & Leibenluft, 2014). They go on to describe it in the following way:

> It [emotion regulation] encompasses the processes that allow the individual to select, attend to, and appraise emotionally arousing stimuli, and to do so flexibly. These processes trigger behavioral and physiological responses that can be modulated in line with goals. Emotion dysregulation arises when these adaptive processes are impaired, leading to behavior that defeats the individual's interests. It encompasses 1) emotional expressions and experiences that are excessive in relation to social norms and are context inappropriate; 2) rapid, poorly controlled shifts in emotion (lability); and 3) the anomalous allocation of attention to emotional stimuli. (Shaw et al., 2014, p. 276)

MBIs are proposed to improve emotion regulation because they teach individuals to observe emotional states as temporary and passing phenomenon that can be responded to in a nonreactive or compassionate manner (Chambers, Gullone, & Allen, 2009; Gratz & Tull, 2010; Guendelman, Medeiros, & Rampes, 2017). Six weeks of MBI training has demonstrated improvements in emotion dysregulation among healthy young adults in comparison to wait-list (Menezes et al., 2013) and active-treatment comparison conditions (Menezes & Bizarro, 2015). As we reviewed in Mitchell et al. (2015), even short-term training has yielded improvements in emotional functioning among healthy meditation novices. For example, a group that received 5 days of meditation training (20 minutes per day) reported improvement on measures of anxiety, depression, anger, and stress-related cortisol in comparison to an active-treatment group (Tang et al., 2007). In another study, those who received 5 weeks of mindfulness training (5–16 minutes per day) exhibited shifts in frontal electroencephalographic asymmetry patterns associated with positive, approach-oriented emotions in comparison to a wait-list group (Moyer et al., 2011).

In terms of biological underpinnings of improved emotion dysregulation in MBIs, one review identified the prefrontal cortex (including dorsal and ventromedial regions), hippocampus, and amygdala as being associated with improvement in emotion regulation after mindfulness training (Hölzel et al., 2011). These regions have also been identified as involved in emotional functioning in individuals diagnosed with ADHD (Barkley, 2010). Overall, given that MBIs improve the ability to regulate emotions and ADHD is a disorder characterized by emotion dysregulation, MBI seems to be an appropriate treatment for ADHD. In addition, although we identify emotion dysregulation and executive functioning as separate mechanisms, one may impact the other. For instance, one model argues that improving executive functioning will have a downstream effect on emotion regulation in MBIs (Teper, Segal, & Inzlicht, 2013).

Impact on Trait Mindfulness

As discussed earlier in this chapter, MBIs are considered to improve mindfulness—the ability to orient attention to the present in the moment, and approach the experience with curiosity, openness, and acceptance. Within the personality literature, mindfulness as a trait is thought to include the following facets: being nonreactive, observing with awareness, acting with awareness, describing with awareness, and adopting a nonjudgmental approach toward one's experience (Baer et al., 2008). Individuals who are low in this trait may be promising candidates for MBIs since this trait is malleable. Those who practice mindfulness meditation may be able to improve this daily expression of mindfulness, thereby improving clinical outcomes.

In a study of 105 adults, half with and half without ADHD, who completed a self-reported trait mindfulness scale, those with ADHD reported lower overall levels of trait mindfulness, particularly on the following subscales: Describing, Acting in Awareness, and Accepting without Judgment (Smalley et al., 2009). Additional analyses indicated that ADHD and trait mindfulness were inversely associated in this study. For example, in a regression predicting trait mindfulness total scores, ADHD group status accounted for a significant portion of variance (16%) after partialing the effects of demographic variables such as age, sex, ethnicity, and education. In another study of adults with and without ADHD, similar findings emerged in which ADHD symptoms were inversely associated with trait mindfulness (Keith, Blackwood, Mathew, & Lecci, 2017). This relationship between ADHD symptoms and trait mindfulness has a strong genetic basis (Siebelink et al., 2019). Given this relationship between ADHD and mindfulness, the use of MBIs in this condition is compelling.

Need for Treatment Options among Adults with ADHD

There is a continuing need for increased treatment options for adults diagnosed with ADHD. Although stimulants are effective in reducing ADHD symptoms, 20–50% are nonresponders and, among those who do respond, adults with ADHD exhibit 50% or less ADHD symptom reduction (Safren, Sprich, Cooper-Vince, Knouse, & Lerner, 2010; Spencer, Biederman, Wilens, & Faraone, 1998; Wilens, Biederman, & Spencer, 1998; Wilens, Spencer, & Biederman, 2002). Among nonpharmacological treatment options, cognitive-behavioral therapy (CBT) is efficacious for ADHD in adulthood (Knouse, Teller, & Brooks, 2017; Young, Moghaddam, & Tickle, 2020). However, there is an unmet patient need—individuals with ADHD and others who want alternative or complementary treatment approaches (Cheung et al., 2015; Hall et al., 2013; Matheson et al., 2013; Swift et al., 2013). In one study that included multicomponent skills training (group DBT, which includes some formal mindfulness techniques) was delivered in an adult ADHD sample, mindfulness was endorsed by 73.8% of the sample as one of the most effective features of the treatment—this aspect of treatment was the second most frequently rated effective treatment component by patients (Philipsen et al., 2007).

Therefore, having treatment options that address patients' identified needs also justifies consideration of treatments such as MBIs.

CURRENT TREATMENT STUDIES OF MBIs FOR ADULTS WITH ADHD

There is growing treatment outcome literature on MBIs to treat ADHD that has been reported on in multiple reviews and meta-analyses (Aadil, Cosme, & Chernaik, 2017; Bachmann et al., 2016; Baijal & Gupta, 2008; Black, Milam, & Sussman, 2009; Cassone, 2015; Davis & Mitchell, 2020; Evans et al., 2018; Krisanaprakornkit, Ngamjarus, Witoonchart, & Piyavhatkul, 2010; Lee et al., 2017; Mitchell et al., 2015; Modesto-Lowe, Farahmand, Chaplin, & Sarro, 2015; Mukerji Househam & Solanto, 2016; Poissant, Mendrek, Talbot, Khoury, & Nolan, 2019; Searight, Robertson, Smith, Perkins, & Searight, 2012; Xue, Zhang, & Huang, 2019; Zhang, Diaz-Roman, & Cortese, 2018). In one recent meta-analysis, MBIs outperform wait-list control conditions and yield medium to large effect sizes for core ADHD symptoms (i.e., Cohen's $d = 0.91$ for inattention, 0.68 for hyperactivity-impulsivity; Cairncross & Miller, 2016). While MBI and ADHD treatment studies include children, adolescents, and adults, the adult literature is particularly developed in respect to the number of treatment studies and methodologies (e.g., randomization and between-group designs).

Table 2.1 provides a summary of peer-reviewed MBI studies targeting adults with ADHD conducted to date. These treatment studies include three that adopted a within-subjects design (Hepark, Kan, & Speckens, 2014; Janssen, de Vries, Hepark, & Speckens, 2020; Zylowska et al., 2008, 2009) and eight that adopted a between-subjects design (Bueno et al., 2015; Edel, Holter, Wassink, & Juckel, 2017; Gu, Xu, & Zhu, 2016; Hepark et al., 2019; Hoxhaj et al., 2018; Janssen et al., 2019; Mitchell et al., 2017; Schoenberg et al., 2014). Notably, one of the between-subjects design studies involved a subset (Schoenberg et al., 2014) of a larger sample (Hepark et al., 2019).

The majority of the above studies have adopted one of two treatment models: a modified MBCT (mMBCT) or MAPs for ADHD. Although the treatments differ in aspects such as number of sessions, both are informed by MBSR (Kabat-Zinn, 1990) and MBCT (Segal et al., 2002) and share points of overlap. Therefore, although these are separate treatments by name, they are not mutually exclusive from one another and instead significantly overlap with one another. Session duration ranged from 6 sessions (Gu et al., 2018) to 13 sessions (Edel et al., 2017) across studies. All but one of these trials (i.e., Gu et al., 2018) administered a MBI in a group therapy format. In addition, all but one of these trials included adult samples diagnosed with ADHD—Zylowska et al. (2008) included adolescents in their sample as well.

Feasibility and Acceptability

Feasibility and acceptability are defined in different ways. In many cases feasibility is assessed by variables such as treatment completion (or, conversely, attrition) rates and session attendance, whereas acceptability is assessed by variables such as treatment satisfaction ratings. In terms of treatment completion, what defined completion varied across studies, such as attending 50% or more of sessions (Hepark et al., 2019; Janssen et

TABLE 2.1. Treatment Outcome Studies of Mindfulness-Based Interventions for Adults with ADHD

Study	Treatment condition	Control condition	Treatment randomization	Assessments	Outcome measures	Main findings [d]
Zylowska et al. (2008, 2009)	MAPs (n = 32)	—	n/a	Pretreatment Posttreatment 3-month follow-up	ADHD-RS/SNAP, BDI/CDI, BAI/RCMAS, ANT, Stroop, Digit Span, Trail Making Test, Vocabulary WAIS/WISC subtest	**ADHD symptoms** (post, 3-month: ADHD-RS/SNAP-IV) **Conflict Detection** (post: ANT) **Depression** (post, 3-month: BDI/CDI) **Anxiety** (post, 3-month: BAI/RCMAS) **Stroop color-word** (post) **Trails A & B** (post: Trail Making Test)
Hepark et al. (2014)	mMBCT (n = 11)	—	n/a	Pretreatment Posttreatment	CAARS-S:SV, BDI-II, KIMS, OQ, STAI, ANT	**ADHD symptoms** (CAARS-S:SV) **Conflict Detection** (ANT) **Mindfulness** (KIMS) **Quality of Life** (OQ)
Janssen et al. (2020)	mMBCT (n = 31)	—	n/a	Pretreatment Posttreatment	CAARS-S:SV, BRIEF, FFMQ-SF, SCS-SF, OQ, HS-SF	**ADHD symptoms** (CAARS-S:SV) **Executive Functioning** (BRIEF) **Self-Compassion** (SCS-SF) **Mental Health Status** (HS-SF)
Mitchell et al. (2017)	MAPs (n = 11)	WL (n = 9)	Yes	Pretreatment Posttreatment	CSS, BRIEF, DEFS, DERS, DTS, ANT, CPT, TMT, DS	**ADHD symptoms** [CSS (self, interview, EMA)] **Executive Functioning** [BRIEF (self, EMA); DEFS (self, interview, EMA)] **Emotion Dysregulation** (DERS, DTS)
Bueno et al. (2015)	MAPs (n = 21)	WL (n = 22)	No	Pretreatment Posttreatment	ASRS, STAI-T, PANAS-X, AAQoL, ANT, CPT	**ADHD symptoms** (ASRS) **Depression** (BDI) **Anxiety** (STAI) **Positive and Negative Affect** (PANAS) **Attention** (CPT Comm. errors and detectability, ANT Hit RT block change)
Schoenberg et al. (2014)	mMBCT (n = 26)	WL (n = 24)	Yes	Pretreatment Posttreatment	CAARS, OQ, KIMS	**ADHD symptoms** (CAARS) **Mindfulness** (KIMS) **Quality of Life** (OQ 45.2)
Hepark et al. (2019)	mMBCT (n = 55)	WL (n = 48)	Yes	Pretreatment Posttreatment	CAARS, OQ, KIMS, BRIEF, BDI-II, STAI,	**ADHD symptoms** [CAARS (self, interview)] **Executive Functioning** (BRIEF)

						Mindfulness (KIMS)
Gu et al. (2018)	mMBCT ($n = 28$)	WL ($n = 26$)	Yes	Pretreatment Posttreatment 3-month follow-up	CAARS, BAI, BDI-II, GPA, MAAS, ANT	**ADHD symptoms** (post, 3 month: CAARS) **Mindfulness** (post, 3 month: MAAS) **Attention** (post, 3 month: ANT Alerting and Orienting RT and error scores) **Depression** (post: BDI-II) **Anxiety** (post: BAI)
Edel et al. (2017)	MBTG ($n = 39$)	DBT ($n = 52$)	No	Pretreatment Posttreatment	WRI, ADHD rating (self, other), MAAS, GSES	—
Hoxhaj et al. (2018)[a]	MAPs ($n = 39$)	PE ($n = 36$)	Yes	Pretreatment Posttreatment 6-month follow-up	CAARS,[b] BDI, SF-36, FFMQ	**Mindfulness** (post: FFMQ Observation and Nonreactivity subscales)
Janssen et al. (2019)[c]	mMBCT + TAU ($n = 52$)	TAU ($n = 55$)	Yes	Pretreatment Posttreatment 3-month follow-up 6-month follow-up	CAARS-INV:SV, CAARS-S:SV, BRIEF, FFMQ-SF, SCS-SF, MHC-SF, OQ	**ADHD symptoms** (post, 3-month, 6-month: CAARS-INV:SV, CAARS-S:SV) **Mindfulness** (post, 3-month, 6-month: FFMQ-SF) **Self-Compassion** (post, 3-month, 6-month: SCS-SF) **Positive Mental Health** (post, 3-month, 6-month: MHC-SF)

Note. Bueno et al. (2015) also included 17 healthy controls. AAQoL = Adult ADHD Quality of Life Questionnaire; ADHD-RS = ADHD Rating Scale—IV (self-report); ANT = Attention Network Task; ASRS = Adult ADHD Self-Report Scale; BAI = Beck Anxiety Inventory; BDI/BDI-II = Beck Depression Inventory; BRIEF = Behavior Rating Inventory of Executive Function (self-report, ecological momentary assessment); BSI = Brief Symptom Inventory; CAARS = Conners' Adult ADHD Rating Scale; CAARS-INV:SV = Conners' Adult ADHD Rating Scale Investigator-Rated Screening Version; CAARS-S:SV = Conners' Adult ADHD Rating Scale—Self Report Short Version; CDI = Children's Depression Inventory; CPT = Conners' Continuous Performance Test; CSS = Current Symptoms Scale (self-report, clinician, ecological momentary assessment); DEFS = Deficits in Executive Functioning Scale (self-report, clinician, ecological momentary assessment); DS = Digit Span; DERS = Difficulties in Emotion Regulation Scale; DTS = Distress Tolerance Scale; GPA = grade point average (official transcript, academic quarter); FFMQ = Five Facet Mindfulness Questionnaire; FFMQ-SF = Five Facet Mindfulness Questionnaire—Short Form; GSES = Generalized Self-Efficacy Scale; HS-SF = Health Status—Short Form; KIMS = Kentucky Inventory of Mindfulness Skills; OQ = Outcome Questionnaire; MAAS = Mindful Attention Awareness Scale; MHC-SF = Mental Health Continuum—Short Form; PANAS-X = Positive and Negative Affect Schedule—Expanded; PE = psychoeducation for ADHD; RCMAS = Revised Children's Manifest Anxiety Scale; SCS-SF = Self-Compassion Scale—Short Form; SF-36 = Short Form Health Survey (36 items); SNAP = Swanson, Nolan, and Pelham Scale IV (self-report); STAI = State–Trait Anxiety Inventory; TAU = treatment as usual; TMT = Trail Making Test; WAIS = Wechsler Adult Intelligence Scale—Revised; WISC = Wechsler Intelligence Scale for Children—Third Edition; WL = wait list; WRI = Wender-Reimherr Interview.

[a]Sample size for each analysis varied at posttreatment (MAPs $n = 39$, PE $n = 36$) and 6 months posttreatment (MAPs $n = 32$, PE $n = 32$).

[b]A blind observer CAARS from a study team assessor was administered as the primary outcome measure, whereas the CAARS observer and self versions were administered as secondary outcome measures.

[c]Sample size based on intent-to-treat analysis at posttreatment, which are the primary findings we report on here. Sample size at 3-month follow-up was 49 (mMBCT + TAU) and 53 (TAU), and at 6-month follow-up was 50 (mMBCT + TAU) and 52 (TAU).

[d]This column lists statistically significant findings that indicated support for the mindfulness-based intervention tested in each respective study.

al., 2020; Zylowska et al., 2008) or 75% or more of sessions (Mitchell et al., 2017). Despite this difference, most who began a MBI for ADHD completed treatment. All studies reported treatment completion that ranged from 73% (Hepark et al., 2014) to 100% (Edel et al., 2017; Mitchell et al., 2017).

The majority of additional feasibility and acceptability findings were reported in trials administering MAPs (Bueno et al., 2015; Mitchell et al., 2017; Zylowska et al., 2008), with a notable exception of an mMBCT study that provided a comprehensive qualitative analysis to investigate barriers/facilitators of participation and processes of change (Janssen et al., 2020).

In MAPs studies, the average number of sessions attended for an eight-session protocol was seven (Mitchell et al., 2017; Zylowska et al., 2008). In Zylowska et al. (2008), the adult sample engaged in 90.3 minutes per week of at-home meditation practice (*SD* = 57.9, weekly averages for the sample ranged from 10.3 minutes to 194.4 minutes). The adult sample engaged in a meditation practice an average of 4.9 days per week (*SD* = 1.6, range = 1.5 to 7.0). Mitchell et al. (2017) conducted weekly clinician session ratings for each subject on a scale of 1 to 5 (higher scores indicating greater adherence) and reported an average at-home exercise adherence of 3.9 (*SD* = 0.36). Bueno et al. (2015) provided group averages of at-home exercises session by session, which ranged from 19.8 minutes (*SD* = 14.1) to 52.9 minutes (*SD* = 48.8).

Treatment satisfaction ratings were also positive. Using a scale ranging from 1 to 10 with higher scores indicating greater overall treatment satisfaction, study participants reported group averages of 9.40 (*SD* = 0.80; Zylowska et al., 2008) and 9.3 (*SD* = 0.90; Bueno et al., 2015). On a similar scale that ranged from 1 to 7, overall treatment satisfaction was 5.91 (*SD* = 1.14; Mitchell et al., 2017). Mitchell et al. also reported that on a scale ranging from 1 (*not at all*) to 4 (*extremely*), participants reported that they learned more about ADHD (*M* = 3.27, *SD* = 0.91); the content they learned was relevant to their experiences (*M* = 3.55, *SD* = 0.93); the techniques/strategies introduced were understandable (*M* = 3.82, *SD* = 0.41); they were confident about regularly using the techniques taught (*M* = 3.36, *SD* = 0.67); and they would recommend mindfulness training to other adults with ADHD (*M* = 3.64, *SD* = 0.92).

Treatment Outcomes: ADHD Symptoms

Across all but two of the studies listed in Table 2.1, inattentive and hyperactive-impulsive ADHD symptoms improved at posttreatment. One of the two exceptions included a trial in which a MBI was compared against a modified DBT group intervention (Edel et al., 2017). There were no differences between these two groups. These null results are important to interpret in the context of a MBI being compared against an intervention that also included mindfulness training, in addition to cognitive-behavioral strategies.[1] Given that CBT is an efficacious intervention for ADHD in adulthood (Knouse et al., 2017; Young et al., 2016), these findings indicate that a MBI is performing as well as an empirically supported psychosocial intervention for ADHD in adults. In the other study that yielded null results, a group that received MAPs and a group that received an ADHD psychoeducation intervention similarly improved in reduction in ADHD symp-

[1] DBT is an intervention that includes CBT strategies.

toms according to blind assessments (Hoxhaj et al., 2018). Notably, the only CBT trial for ADHD in adulthood that yielded null results in which both groups improved was an ADHD psychoeducation intervention as the treatment comparison condition (Vidal et al., 2013). Therefore, the mindfulness intervention performed just as well as an active-treatment comparison that performs just as well as the most empirically supported non-medication treatment for ADHD in adulthood.

Across the remaining studies that supported the efficacy of mindfulness for ADHD, three conducted assessments beyond posttreatment (Gu et al., 2018; Janssen et al., 2019; Zylowska et al., 2009). All three studies reported maintained improvement in ADHD symptoms—these studies included a within-group design in comparison to pretreatment scores (Zylowska et al., 2009), a between-group design in comparison to a wait-list control condition (Gu et al., 2018), and a between-group design in comparison to a treatment-as-usual condition (Janssen et al., 2019). Overall, across all of these studies supporting that a MBI improved ADHD symptoms, reporting sources varied. For example, some studies included self-report only (Bueno et al., 2015; Gu et al., 2018; Hepark et al., 2014; Janssen et al., 2020; Schoenberg et al., 2014; Zylowska et al., 2008), while others incorporated clinician assessments (Edel et al., 2017; Hepark et al., 2019; Mitchell et al., 2017). One of the largest trials to date included a blinded rater and indicated that ADHD symptoms improved for the MBI group in comparison to a treatment-as-usual group (Janssen et al., 2019). One study also included ecological momentary assessment, which involved participants providing "in-the-moment" ratings of symptoms outside of a clinic or laboratory setting in their daily lives (Mitchell et al., 2017). These findings indicated that ADHD symptoms rated using this method indicated improvement for a MBI group relative to a wait-list comparison group.

Some studies also reported the proportion of study participants with 30% or more symptom reduction (Figure 2.1), which is considered a measure of clinical significance. Proportions ranged from 26% (Janssen et al., 2020) to 71% (Gu et al., 2018) when ADHD symptoms were assessed via self-report. Across these studies, the overall average proportion of participants who endorsed 30% or more ADHD symptom improvement was 49%. Similarly, proportions ranged from 27% (Janssen et al., 2019) to 72% (Mitchell et al., 2017) for clinician ratings. Across these studies, the overall average proportion of participants who endorsed 30% or more ADHD symptom improvement was 43%. One study used ecological momentary assessments to measure ADHD symptoms reported that 27% of the sample improved using this assessment approach (Mitchell et al., 2017).

Treatment Outcomes: Executive Functions

Another variable that was widely considered across the studies listed in Table 2.1 was executive functioning, including assessment using self-report, clinician ratings, ecological momentary assessment, and laboratory task performance. Self-reported executive functioning was primarily assessed using the adult version of the Behavior Rating Inventory of Executive Functioning (BRIEF; Roth, Isquith, & Gioia, 2005). The BRIEF yields an overall total score that is composed of two index scores, the Behavioral Regulation Index and the Metacognitive Index. The Behavioral Regulation Index includes four subscales (Inhibit, Shift, Emotional Control, and Self-Monitor), and the Metacognitive Index includes five subscales (Initiate, Working Memory, Plan/Organize,

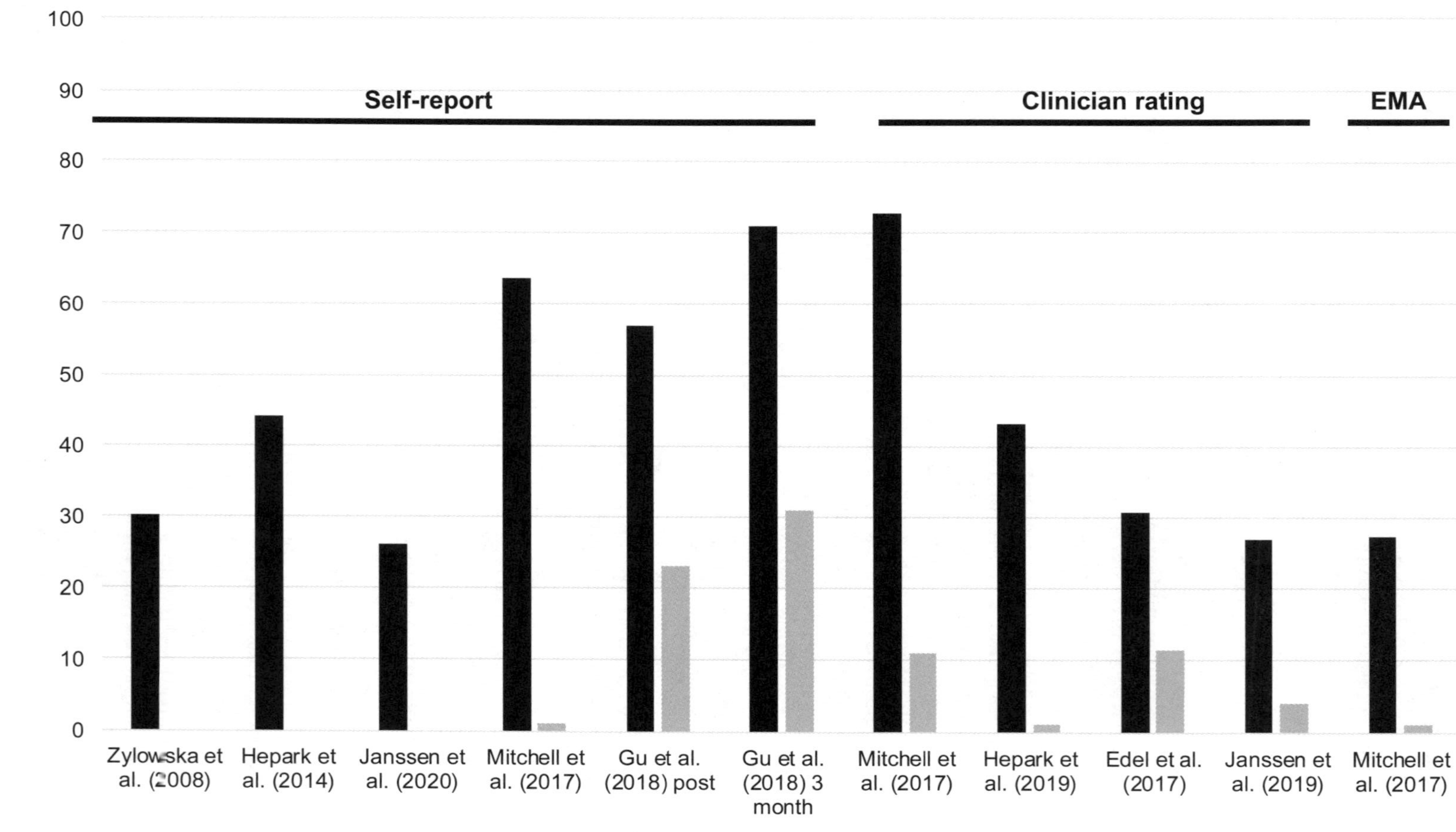

FIGURE 2.1. Proportion of study participants with 30% or more symptom reduction across three different methods of assessment (self-report, clinician ratings, and ecological momentary assessment [EMA]) in MBI adult ADHD treatment-outcome studies.

Task Monitor, and Organization of Materials). Across studies that used the BRIEF or other self-report executive-functioning measures, total score or subscale scores significantly improved (Hepark et al., 2019; Janssen et al., 2020; Mitchell et al., 2017) with one exception. In Janssen et al. (2019), BRIEF scores were not different between groups at posttreatment. However, group differences that indicated more improvement for the mindfulness treatment group emerged over the follow-up assessment period. Clinician ratings were assessed in one study using the Deficits in Executive Functioning Scale (Barkley, 2011b). In this study (Mitchell et al., 2017), executive functioning significantly improved in the MBI treatment condition across assessments in comparison to the wait-list control group with large effect sizes. The same study was also the only one to utilize ecological momentary assessment and similarly reported improvements "in-the-moment" when executive-functioning behaviors were assessed in the natural environment. For laboratory task performance, four of the studies utilized different testing batteries (Bueno et al., 2015; Gu et al., 2018; Mitchell et al., 2017; Zylowska et al., 2008), though all included the Attention Network Task (Fan & Posner, 2004). Executive functioning improved on at least one measure across these studies with one exception (i.e., Mitchell et al., 2017). However, the null results in Mitchell et al. (2017) may have been a function of a lack of a stimulant medication washout period for those prescribed medication for ADHD. When medication washout periods were utilized, improvements were observed in studies adopting a within-subjects design (Zylowska et al., 2008) and a between-subjects design (Bueno et al., 2015).

Treatment Outcomes: Emotional Functioning

Consistent with the proposals that adult patients with ADHD are responsive to MBIs due to their effects on emotion dysregulation, one hypothesis is that emotion dysregulation should be improved at posttreatment. More broadly, aspects of emotional functioning may improve. However, the research results are mixed: measures of emotional functioning (i.e., depressed mood, anxiety) improved in some studies (Bueno et al., 2015; Gu et al., 2018; Zylowska et al., 2008), but not in others (Hepark et al., 2014, 2019; Hoxhaj et al., 2018). In the only study that assessed emotion dysregulation directly via two self-report measures to assess the construct, the ADHD group reported significantly greater improvement with larger effect sizes over time in comparison to a wait-list comparison group (Mitchell et al., 2017).

Treatment Outcomes: Trait Mindfulness and Other Functional Outcomes

Additional constructs regularly examined in existing treatment outcome studies are improvement in trait mindfulness and functional outcomes such as quality of life. Regarding trait mindfulness, total or subscale scores improved in six trials (Gu et al., 2018; Hepark et al., 2014, 2019; Hoxhaj et al., 2018; Janssen et al., 2019; Schoenberg et al., 2014), but not one (Janssen et al., 2020). Other functional outcomes (e.g., self-compassion) and quality of life improved on at least one measure in some studies (Hepark et al., 2014; Janssen et al., 2019, 2020; Schoenberg et al., 2014), but not others (Bueno et al., 2015; Hepark et al., 2019; Hoxhaj et al., 2018).

Overall, across these studies, ADHD symptoms improved, as well as executive functioning and trait mindfulness. Emotion dysregulation, emotional functioning (i.e., anxiety and depression), and functional outcomes/quality of life may also have improved, but more research is needed in these areas due to limited and mixed results. Larger samples to increase statistical power to identify treatment effects, greater use of blinded raters, correction for multiple comparisons among a large number of outcome measures, and follow-up periods beyond 3 months are needed in future studies. In addition, factors that could impact outcomes, such as treatment adherence, should be considered. Finally, neuroplastic changes via neuroimaging and medication effects should be investigated as well. On the whole, despite the need for further research, the available studies, particularly three trials of MAPs, demonstrate that MBIs improve ADHD symptoms among adults with the disorder.

Other Peer-Reviewed MAPs Trials

One other study not reviewed above that examined the MAPs intervention was conducted in a female adolescent sample with elevated ADHD symptoms (Kiani, Hadianfard, & Mitchell, 2017). This study included a MAPs treatment group (n = 15) against a wait-list comparison group (n = 15). A self-report measure of emotion dysregulation and executive-functioning laboratory task performance were considered as outcome variables. Those in the treatment group reported improvement in emotion dysregulation in comparison to the wait-list control group at posttreatment with large effect sizes. In terms of executive functioning task performance, planning and inhibition improved in the treatment group relative to the control group with large effect sizes at posttreatment.

SUMMARY

This chapter reviews MBIs and their application in ADHD. Given the self-regulation mechanisms that MBIs are purported to impact, such as attentional/executive functioning, emotion dysregulation, and trait mindfulness, ADHD is a particularly promising target for this intervention. Treatment outcome studies of adults with ADHD indicate that the treatment is feasible and acceptable. MBIs, particularly MAPs, have demonstrated improvements in core symptoms of the disorder as well as characteristic features of the disorder, such as executive functioning and emotion dysregulation.

CHAPTER 3

Teaching Considerations
Common Questions and Answers

In this chapter, we provide a summary of common questions practitioners may have about the MAPs for ADHD Program and answers to provide guidance.

What is your overall teaching philosophy?

The overall teaching philosophy is based on the following intentions: (1) demystify both ADHD and mindfulness; (2) provide a compelling rationale for mindfulness practice in the context of ADHD knowledge; (3) offer a gradual introduction of formal mindfulness exercises (starting with 5-minute practice and building to 15 minutes over 8 weeks); (4) start with practices that train focus and monitoring of attention and later expand to include open-/receptive-attention practices for self-regulation; (5) utilize strategies that support habit formation of mindfulness-based strategies in everyday activities (e.g., reminders or buddy system); (6) use visual aids to enhance learning; and (7) encourage both formal and informal mindfulness practices, and empower each participant to find their own way to practice mindfulness.

Is mindfulness training secular or does it have spiritual or religious connotations?

This question can be on the mind of some therapists new to mindfulness-based therapy or those who first learned mindfulness in a religious context. The question can also come up when discussing this approach with participants, especially those with strong religious or faith backgrounds who are skeptical of mindfulness as either "new age" or in some way interfering with their religious practices.

We want to acknowledge that this is a complex and controversial question, as some would argue that mindfulness cannot or should not be taught without a world view based in Buddhist values and ethics. For more in-depth discussion, see articles discussing various perspectives on this issue (Harrington & Dunne, 2015; Schmidt, 2016;

Thupten, 2018). However, in discussions with participants, we typically emphasize that mindfulness involves attention and awareness exercises that, in the context of therapy, are secular and related to training of cognitive and emotional abilities (i.e., self-regulation). We may point out that while mindfulness evolved in the context of Eastern spiritual traditions such as Buddhism, it is also an approach to studying the human mind and can be taught separately from the spiritual context. We also point out that if desired, the secular mindful awareness skills can be brought to personal faith rituals regardless of what faith the person is practicing.

What format: group or individual? What about online delivery?

The MAPs for ADHD Program was developed primarily for in-person group delivery. The research studies with MAPs for ADHD used a format of eight weekly sessions, each 2–2.5 hours long. In those studies, group size varied from 6 (adults) or 8 (teens) to 24 (adults). In clinical practice, the group size can vary depending on available space and comfort of the mindfulness trainer (MT).[1] In general, we recommend group size to be at least 6–8 patients in size so if there is variability in attendance, the group can still meet with enough members.

While we recommend 2- to 2.5-hour weekly sessions, as this is the evidence-supported length of training, we foresee that some therapists or teachers may wish to shorten the group sessions to 1- or 1.5-hour sessions and/or adjust the length of the course to fit the logistical constraints of their setting or to make it easier for participants to attend. In addition, modifications may also include adapting MAPs for individual in-person therapy or online delivery. These alternative modes of delivery could be beneficial, as studies in other populations have supported efficacy of similarly modified trainings (Galla et al., 2015; Kemper 2017; Lyzwinski, Caffery, Bambling, & Edirippulige, 2018). Additional research in non-ADHD samples suggests that even short-term mindful breath-awareness training for 3 weeks improves inhibitory control and response monitoring (Pozuelos, Mead, Rueda, & Malinowski, 2019). However, it continues to be an open question in terms of what constitutes an adequate amount of training to see meaningful impact on ADHD-related symptoms or impairments. At this time, there is a need for research studies investigating feasibility or effectiveness of shortened sessions, an individual therapy format, or online delivery for adults with ADHD.

Is the group process in MAPs different from other group therapy models?

In teaching mindfulness skills, MTs encourage investigation and trust of one's own direct experience in the present moment. Throughout the training, the MTs model curiosity and facilitate individual discovery of one's direct experiences—body sensations, emotions, thoughts—with openness and without judgment. While some didactic content is offered in the MAPs for ADHD Program, it is preferred that the core principles are explored via experiential exercises and elicited from the participants versus directly explained by the MTs. During the inquiry about their experiences, the participants are guided to reflect on their direct experiences and how they may relate to living with ADHD. During such reflections, the MTs are vigilant for the tendency

[1] We use the term "mindfulness trainer" to describe mental health professionals leading these groups rather than other descriptors (e.g., clinicians or therapists) to emphasize the importance of meditation experience among those who are teaching this program.

participants often have to be caught in "the story" or analysis of why the inner experience is happening. The MTs are also vigilant for their own tendencies to focus on the content and offer solutions, interpretation, or analysis of the experience. If needed, the MTs redirect the participants to notice their direct experience instead of being overly caught up in the interpretation or "the story." For example, MTs might encourage this by asking questions such as, "What body sensations do you notice right now as you talk?" and "What other feelings do you notice in this very moment?" For more discussion on the process and facilitation in mindfulness-based groups, please see *Mindfulness-Based Relapse Prevention for Addictive Behaviors: A Clinician's Guide* (Bowen, Chawla, & Marlatt, 2011).

Why is a group format common with mindfulness-based trainings?

Seminal mindfulness trainings, such as MBSR (Kabat-Zinn, 1982; Kabat-Zinn et al., 1985) and MBCT (Segal et al., 2002), that MAPs and many "next-generation" MBIs are derived from, are typically delivered in a group format for several reasons. The group setting allows for sharing of experiences between patients (e.g., sharing difficulties and successes with meditation practice, common patterns of ADHD, insights gained from the approach) and lends itself better for delivering longer guided meditations (vs. individual therapy). In general, trainings or therapy delivered in group settings help destigmatize one's condition and offer peer support opportunities independent of the type of intervention. In addition, all of the treatment outcome research on the MAPs for ADHD Program has been exclusively conducted using a group format, which is consistent with other mindfulness for ADHD research. However, we realize that some clinicians may want to use a similar approach in individual therapy; therefore, throughout the manual we discuss strategies for adapting the MAPs for ADHD Program to such a context (see the question below).

Of note, the mindfulness-based training for ADHD can be delivered as an educational offering (i.e., a class) or a psychotherapy group. For example, an ADHD coach who is not a clinician may offer this training as a class, in the same way that MBSR groups can be conducted by nonclinicians. A clinician may offer it as a class or a psychotherapy group, depending on his or her experience or preference. The pros and cons to consider are:

1. *Class format.* In addition to those with ADHD, the class may include family members, partners, or interested clinicians. Age requirement may be more liberal, with ages 15 and up attending together, and screening requirements can be less stringent. Location of the group can be in clinical or nonclinical spaces. This can increase access. However, the patients have to pay out-of-pocket for the class fee (i.e., no insurance billing). Also, with less screening or diagnostic evaluation, the mindfulness instructor typically will have less knowledge of who is in the group and less ability to control the composition of the group.
2. *Group psychotherapy format.* Typically there is more oversight of who is in the group through referral or diagnostic evaluation requirements. Insurance billing can be used. Clinical group spaces have to be utilized and appropriate group therapy documentation is needed. The groups are typically smaller (8–12 people), potentially affording the clinician to bring in more personalized and clinical knowledge to the group. The instructor may have dual roles of being

participants' individual clinician (therapist or prescriber) as well as a group therapist.

How do I adapt the training to individual format?

The training can be adapted to individual format by spreading out the content over several additional weeks. This is because most individual sessions are 45 to 60 minutes and because patients may bring up other clinical issues that need to be discussed within the meeting time. Typically, each group session requires two to three individual sessions to cover the main theme and demonstrate one to two experiential exercises. Consequently, if individual sessions are scheduled weekly, the full MAPs for ADHD training may take 3–6 months. Alternatively, a clinician can choose certain elements of MAPs and weave them into the psychotherapy meetings alongside other interventions such as CBT or supportive therapy. As you will see in the session-by-session content, we provide tips to guide practitioners who want to administer the MAPs for ADHD Program in an individual therapy setting.

If elements of MAPs are introduced into an existing psychotherapy relationship, it would be important to prepare the patient for the transition and invite the patient to dialogue about his or her comfort level with the change and the mindfulness exercises. The patient may feel self-conscious being the only one that is guided through an exercise in a session, or may find the periods of silence uncomfortable. Giving patients a choice of either keeping their eyes open (resting in one spot) or closing eyes during meditation can ease the comfort level with meditations in this context. We also find that it's important for therapists to discuss what they will be doing during the exercises and to specifically inquire about how the patient feels about this. If this aspect of the therapist's behavior during the exercises is not explicitly addressed, the ambiguity may insert an additional layer of discomfort for the patient. For example, a patient may wonder if the clinician is going to be staring at them during the exercise. We recommend participating in the exercises yourself while also facilitating the exercise as the therapist. In any case, an open and transparent communication style is necessary. Starting with brief meditation practices and checking in about the experience right after will also ensure that the therapist and the patient are collaborating in taking this new direction in individual therapy.

Another factor to consider is that some practices, such as mindful walking, are not done as easily in an individual session as in a group setting. Thus discussion of the practice and further resources can be given instead of actually practicing it in the session.

Keep in mind that, as we mention above, delivery of the mindfulness training for ADHD in individual format has not been widely researched. Available one-on-one training descriptions often mix mindfulness, CBT, and other supportive strategies. For an example, see *Mindfulness for Teens with ADHD* (Burdick, 2017).

Can MAPs exercises be adapted for individuals with various physical or sensory difficulties?

The mindfulness exercises can and should be creatively adapted for individuals that have unique challenges. For example, individuals with physical limitations (e.g., chronic pain or in a wheelchair) should be guided to practice mindful movement only in a way that is feasible and comfortable for them. Instead of a mindful walking practice, the participants may try gently tapping or pressing their feet into the ground while sitting, and feeling the sensations at the bottom of their feet in this way. If the latter is difficult, the participants may choose to press their palms against their lap as if simulating walking and feel the alternating sensations there. It is important to give participants permission to "listen to your body" or "don't do anything that feels uncomfortable or too much for you." The MT should let patients know that all practices are optional, emphasizing choice and "taking care of yourself" throughout each class. The option of keeping eyes open and resting (vs. closed), or opening eyes when not feeling comfortable during the silent practice, should be offered at the beginning of the course and reiterated at other times in the training, especially if there are participants with a history of trauma. Those with a history of trauma may experience periods of dissociation or flooding with memories during meditation and opening eyes can help re-ground them. If such trauma-related difficulties are happening frequently and/or are significantly distressing, the MT should consider whether group format is best suited for the participant; perhaps individual format and/or different form of therapy is more appropriate. Overall, we encourage MTs to use simple instructions (avoiding long, multistep sentences that may be difficult to process and avoiding jargon), encourage self-pacing that is comfortable (not too slow or too fast) for the participants, and look out for signs of discomfort or distress in any of the participants. If distress is noted yet not proactively shared in the group discussion, the MT should check with the struggling participant during a break or after the class to see if adaptations (e.g., noticing sensations of one's palms resting instead of the breath if focusing on the breath provokes anxiety—something some patients with history of clinical anxiety disorder report) or additional help (e.g., referral for individual therapy) are needed.

What is the difference between MBSR, MBCT, and MAPs for ADHD? I am familiar with the other programs, so can I use MBSR or MBCT for adult ADHD?

MAPs for ADHD is derived from MBSR and MBCT (of note MBCT was also modeled after MBSR), so the programs share many similarities. We developed the MAPs for ADHD approach with the intention to make it more ADHD-friendly than the other programs by including ADHD psychoeducation and breaking down the mindfulness training into steps, making it more gradual (also see the first question, above, regarding teaching philosophy). Formal practice starts with 5 minutes (Sessions 1 and 2), increases to 10 minutes (Sessions 3–5), and then up to 15 minutes (Sessions 6–8). Other notable differences are that (1) while mindful movement is included, yoga poses are deemphasized for ease of delivery and (2) self-compassion is more explicitly included. The overall intention is to make the MAPs training more relevant and accessible for those with ADHD. However, MBCT (often with ADHD education) has also been successfully used with adult ADHD groups and has a growing evidence base (see Chapter 2). Overall, mindfulness instructors trained in the other approaches are well-positioned to deliver MAPs for ADHD.

I have read **The Mindfulness Prescription for Adult ADHD** *book by Dr. Zylowska. How is MAPs for ADHD different from the content there?*

The Mindfulness Prescription for Adult ADHD is a self-help book based on the MAPs for ADHD training (Zylowska, 2012). This book is a clinical manual that includes instructions for delivering this approach. Overall, the principles and the structure outlined in *The Mindfulness Prescription* book are closely related to the MAPs for ADHD Program outlined here, and both books are resources for those interested in this approach. In our groups, we have used *The Mindfulness Prescription* book as a source of audio for guided meditation (see *www.shambhala.com/MindfulnessPrescription*) and an additional participant reference during the MAPs for ADHD training. For each session, we include relevant pages from the book as optional reading (Table 3.1).

Can MAPs for ADHD be used with children or teens with ADHD?

Most research studies on the MAPs for ADHD Program were delivered to adults with ADHD, so the available evidence is most supportive of its use with adults (Cairncross & Miller, 2016; Mitchell et al., 2015; Poissant et al., 2019). However, an initial MAPs for ADHD study tested its feasibility with a group of older teens (15–18 years old, $n = 8$), showing that the training was feasible and showed pre- and postimprovements in ADHD symptoms and selected cognitive measures (Zylowska et al., 2008). A study among female adolescents high in ADHD symptoms similarly provided promising support that MAPs can be administered to teens (Kiani et al., 2017). The MAPs for ADHD training was also piloted with a group of ADHD children 9–12 years old in Australia,

TABLE 3.1. Correspondence between MAPs and *The Mindfulness Prescription for Adult ADHD* Book

MAPs for ADHD	*The Mindfulness Prescription for Adult ADHD* book
1: Introduction to ADHD and Mindfulness.	1: Part I (Extensive introduction to ADHD and Mindfulness), pages 11–54 Step 1 (Attention exercises, 5 Senses including Mindful Eating), pages 55–68
2: Mindful Awareness of ADHD Patterns	2: Mindful Awareness of ADHD Patterns, pages 49–50 Step 2 (Breathing), pages 69–79
3: Sound, Breath, and Body[a]	3: Step 3 (Sound, Breath, and Body), pages 80–88
4: Body Sensations	4: Step 4 (Body Sensations and Movement), pages 9–109
5: Thoughts	5: Step 5 (Thoughts), pages 110–127
6: Emotions	6: Step 6 (Feelings), pages 128–153
7: Presence and Interactions	7: Step 7 (Listening and Speaking), pages 154–168
8: Review, Wrap-Up	8: Step 8 (Decisions and Actions), pages 169–193, and Putting It All Together, pages 194–201

[a]Early version of the MAPs for ADHD training has this session listed as Breath, Body, and Sound. This was subsequently changed as the awareness of sound practice is the first practice of this session.

suggesting that the training can be delivered with beneficial results in this younger population (Uliando, 2010). Other mindfulness-training models have also been tried, such as concurrent parent and child groups from the MYmind program (Bögels, Hoogstad, van Dun, de Schutter, & Restifo, 2008; van de Weijer-Bergsma, Formsma, de Bruin, & Bögels, 2012; van der Oord, Bögels, & Peijnenburg, 2012). However, due to research design limitations (e.g., no control group) and small sample sizes of both such up-to-date studies, more work is needed to understand the utility of this training with children and teens with ADHD (see Davis & Mitchell, 2020, for a review). More methodologically rigorous trials are needed to establish the efficacy of MBIs in children with ADHD and their families (Evans et al., 2018).

Is there a general structure to each MAPs for ADHD session?

Yes, Sessions 2–7 all have the following sequential structure:

1. Short mindfulness practice (usually review of a practice from a prior session)
2. Introduction of a new topic (e.g., mindfulness of emotions) in the context of ADHD
3. Practice of a new guided meditation followed by inquiry (i.e., debriefing how the practice went and what was noticed). Typically two or three new meditations are introduced
4. Discussion of at-home practice, both formal and informal
5. Brief closing appreciation or loving-kindness meditation

Sessions 1 and 8 (the beginning and closing sessions, respectively) have a modified structure to allow for unique topics such as introductions, rationale for treatment, and guidelines for group participation (Session 1) and closing ceremony and resources/tips for continuing practice after the MAPs training is over (Session 8).

What kinds of supplies or other logistical considerations are needed for this group training?

The MT needs the following items:

1. Sign-in sheet
2. Chairs and/or meditation cushions
3. Meditation bell
4. Handouts for at-home practice and/or to enhance learning
5. Whiteboard to highlight information in a visual way
6. Clock, watch, or timer to help with time management during each session
7. Any assessment materials to track treatment progress (e.g., ADHD symptoms)
8. Raisins or other food for mindful eating (Session 1)
9. Ability to play music (Session 3)
10. Closing ceremony items (Session 8)

The training space should be large enough to accommodate at least six people (sitting in a circle is ideal). Outdoor or indoor space large enough to allow for mindful walking exercise is also recommended. Other aspects that trainers may want to consider include provision of session-by-session binders that contain all treatment handouts, an agenda for each session, and a setting that minimizes distractions (e.g., sounds from a busy hallway).

Is there a website where I can download handouts or guided meditations for the participants?

Enlarged versions of the book's handouts and examples of recorded guided meditations can be downloaded from The Guilford Press website (see the box at the end of the table of contents).

What participant characteristics or cautions should I consider before offering the training?

The MAPs for ADHD Program was developed and tested among adults with an ADHD diagnosis following current *Diagnostic and Statistical Manual of Mental Disorders* (DSM) criteria (American Psychiatric Association, 2013) (described in more detail in Chapter 4). Ideally, all group participants should have received an ADHD diagnosis following empirically based assessment guidelines prior to receiving this intervention. As part of a comprehensive assessment for ADHD, participant comorbid psychiatric conditions should have also been taken into account. In general, significant mood symptoms (moderate to severe depression, hypomania or mania), ongoing substance use, severe personality disorder that may interfere with group delivery, psychotic symptoms, and recent history of trauma are considered contraindications to mindfulness-based treatment (Van Dam et al., 2018). Of note, mindfulness training has been studied and found promising for treatment of substance use relapse prevention, chronic schizophrenia, and posttraumatic stress disorder; however, those trainings have their own adaptations and specifications that are not included in the MAPs for ADHD Program. In general, individual sessions with treatment protocols designed for these clinical features are better suited for these patients. See Mitchell, Bates, and Zylowska (2018) for an overview of potential adverse events to consider for people with ADHD.

In addition, a screening prior to treatment should be conducted to ensure that the goals of this treatment align with the goals of the participant. Participants' active interest in a mindfulness approach may predict better engagement and response. Research studies in depression have shown that matching patients' preferences with given treatment improves attendance and outcomes (Kwan, Dimidjian, & Rizvi, 2010). Consequently, patients who don't show an interest in mindfulness as a treatment for ADHD in adulthood may not be good candidates. Alternatively, their motivation to "try something new" can be assessed and the therapist can ask if they're willing to "give mindfulness a shot."

How are any major issues of nonadherence or dropout managed in the group?

Premature discontinuation of therapy, or dropping out, is a common phenomenon across therapy formats and orientation, and discontinuation is estimated to be between

20 and 30% across studies (Ogrodniczuk, Joyce, & Piper, 2005; Swift & Greenberg, 2012). Strategies commonly used to mitigate this problem include adequate screening and patient selection prior to treatment initiation, appointment reminders, motivation enhancement, and good therapeutic alliance. In our experience, the following can be helpful: (1) acknowledging in the group that missing sessions can happen and encouraging participants to return even if they missed a session or two (e.g., "even if you fall off the wagon, you can always get back on"); (2) reaching out to patients who did not show up and inviting them back; (3) sending out a summary at-home practice to those who have missed a session; and (4) checking in individually during a break or after a session with those who missed a session. If MTs notice that someone is nonadherent during the group (e.g., not participating in an exercise), the MTs can use their discretion whether to address this in a group or individually. We recommend modeling curiosity and nonjudgmental perspective in asking the participants something along these lines: "I noticed you were not participating. Can you share with us what happened for you during the last exercise?" Disruptive behaviors such as too much talking, inappropriate sharing, or frankly disruptive behavior should be addressed by redirecting the person in the group, pulling them aside, and/or, if needed, terminating from the group while giving a referral to another treatment option.

I work with a specific subgroup within adult ADHD (e.g., women or college students). Are there any special considerations for delivering MAPs for ADHD with such populations?

Having a mindfulness-based training within a group that shares similar concerns can create more cohesion and invite specific delivery considerations or topics to discuss. As many women are primary caregivers to children, finding time for themselves often involves arranging childcare. Offering childcare during the course of the MAPs training or, alternatively, offering concurrent child and mother mindfulness groups could improve access. Similarly, an online mindfulness group can be popular and easier to attend for women working both at home and outside the home. Topics such as (1) challenges of motherhood, especially if children also have ADHD; (2) impact of hormonal fluctuations and perimenopause on ADHD symptoms; and (3) finding balance and time for self-care should be woven into the psychoeducation and group discussion. Kathleen Nadeau, an expert in the area of women and ADHD, has noted that

> while a group for women needs to gently help them become more self-focused and able to meet their own needs, we've found that it's almost impossible not to talk about the challenges of motherhood with ADHD kids, but also just about the practicalities of finding time for uninterrupted mindfulness—whether in a group class or in individual mindfulness practice . . . almost all moms are overcommitted, between work, family life, household management, and kids after school activities. Helping them to find a better balance and to be more realistic about what they can reasonably expect of themselves is so critical to helping women with ADHD to function better. (personal communication)

Similarly, working with college students, one has to consider the unique needs of this group. Delivering MAPs for ADHD training at or in collaboration with campus' counseling and psychological services and disability resource centers (where many

ADHD students seek educational accommodations) can help with recruitment and accessibility. Common topics to include are developing ADHD-friendly study skills, optimizing one's learning style, time management, and dealing with performance or test anxiety. Establishing and maintaining healthy daily routines and habits (such as regular sleeping or eating) should be emphasized. The topic of risks of substance abuse or overusing stimulants to study (by students with or without ADHD) may also come up in this group. Finally, connecting new students to appropriate supports such as disability resource sources or tutoring and learning self-advocacy with college instructors should be woven into the discussion. In this more digitally native group, connection to each other via text or group app (such as WhatsApp) can arise spontaneously or be more easily adopted when suggested by the instructor. As other learning differences may be present in addition to ADHD, such as dyslexia or dyspraxia, presenting MAPs for ADHD along with study skills and in a multisensory way can be helpful. Such an approach has been used by a team of learning-disorders specialists—Karis Krcmar and Tina Horsman from the United Kingdom—in their book *Mindfulness for Study: From Procrastination to Action* (2016). The resource includes chapters about reading for successful study, effective writing for academic purposes, revision and exam strategies, and mindful use of the internet.

How much knowledge of ADHD should I have to teach this approach?

We recommend having sufficient knowledge of adult ADHD symptoms and associated impairments to effectively impart ADHD education and answer any questions that may arise in the group. Participants may have heard previous inaccurate information about ADHD or have questions related to their lived experience with ADHD, and the therapist should be very comfortable handling such discussion. The therapist should also understand how ADHD-related challenges can influence one's engagement with the mindfulness training and use strategies informed by the broader ADHD knowledge to support the participants.

The basic knowledge includes DSM diagnostic criteria (American Psychiatric Association, 2013), including symptom count, childhood onset, pervasiveness, and symptom impact on daily living. In Chapter 4 we discuss the core ADHD psychoeducation and how it can be presented it in the context of MAPs for ADHD.

How does this treatment approach fit within other adult ADHD treatment options?

A multimodal approach to treatment (i.e., pharmacotherapy and psychosocial treatment) is generally recommended for adult ADHD. We typically discuss with patients what their ADHD treatment options are and how MBIs can complement them. We describe to patients how medications (mainly stimulants) and CBT are efficacious for ADHD in adulthood (De Crescenzo, Cortese, Adamo, & Janiri, 2017; Young et al., 2016). We also highlight that MBIs are shown to be feasible and acceptable for adults with ADHD, and have increasing support for efficacy (see Chapter 2). This dialogue may also include consideration of treatment targets, which may influence patient preferences. For example, while the MAPs intervention has been shown to improve emotion dysregulation in adults with ADHD (see Chapter 2), CBT for adults with ADHD has not.

The therapist can also discuss with patients what CBT and MBIs have in common and their points of difference (see Mitchell et al., 2015, for a discussion). In general we think CBT and mindfulness training can complement each other well and are well suited for combining. As stated above, we always consider a patient's preference and unless the treatment literature contraindicates their preference, the treatment(s) are selected collaboratively. As a general rule, the therapist should be careful not to jeopardize the treatment alliance by trying too hard to convince the patient of the validity of a particular treatment, while also making the current "state of the science" for treatment clear. One way to accomplish this is for the therapist to have a strong knowledge of the treatment literature for ADHD, balanced with understanding patient preferences and needs.

How much mindfulness practice do I have to do personally to teach this approach?

Unlike other psychotherapy approaches, it is recommended that the MTs have been through mindfulness training themselves and have an ongoing mindfulness practice (formal and/or informal practice). The professional guidelines as to intensity of prior mindfulness training to be an effective MT have not yet been established; however, participation in recognized mindfulness teacher certification programs such as MBCT or MBSR is strongly recommended. Overall, it is widely recognized that significant experiential knowledge (e.g., understanding the difficulties of sitting practice and insights into the inner dynamic while meditating) that can only be gained by actual practice is crucial for effective teaching.

What measures can I use to assess patients' responses to the training?

Response to the training can be assessed using measures of engagement as well as measures of outcomes:

1. Participants' weekly attendance and the at-home practice records (see Handouts in the Appendix) are used to assess engagement with mindfulness practice. Electronic means of logging practice may also be explored via smartphone applications.
2. To assess outcomes, see a comprehensive review of available assessment tools in adults with ADHD (Ramsay, 2017). Additional measures used in mindfulness research can capture changes expected to correlate with mindfulness-based treatment mechanisms and outcomes. Here is a selected list of measures previously used in adult ADHD and/or mindfulness research:
    - *ADHD symptoms.* Scales such as the Current Symptoms Scale (Barkley & Murphy, 2006), adapted to measure symptoms over the past 7 days; the Conners' Adult ADHD Rating Scale (Conners, Erhardt, & Sparrow, 1999); or the Barkley Adult ADHD Rating Scale (Barkley, 2011a). A commonality across these measures is that they include DSM-based ADHD symptoms.
    - *Executive functions.* The Behavior Rating Inventory of Executive Functioning—Adult Version (Roth et al., 2005; Roth, Lance, Isquith, Fischer, & Giancola, 2013) and the Deficits in Executive Functioning Scale (Barkley, 2011b) are self-report rating scales (the latter scale also has a clinician interview format), whereas

the Conners' Continuous Performance Test (Conners, 1995) and Attention Network Task (Fan & Posner, 2004) are commonly used laboratory tasks.

- *Emotional functioning.* The Beck Depression Inventory (Beck & Steer, 1984; Beck et al., 1961) and Beck Anxiety Inventory (Beck et al., 1988) may be administered for mood states, whereas measures such as the Difficulties in Emotion Regulation Scale (Gratz & Roemer, 2004) may be administered to assess how well such mood states are regulated.
- *Mindfulness.* The Mindful Attention Awareness Scale (Brown & Ryan, 2003) and the Five Facet Mindfulness Questionnaire (Baer et al., 2008) are often used to measure trait mindfulness.
- *Well-being.* The Self-Compassion Scale—Short Form (Raes, Pommier, Neff, & Van Gucht, 2011) or the Perceived Stress Scale (Cohen, Kamarck, & Mermelstein, 1983).

Those who are interested in additional measures such as measures of attention, working memory, mind wandering, or impulsivity should consult measures often used in the research literature, such as the studies discussed in Chapter 2.

CHAPTER 4

ADHD Psychoeducation

In this chapter, we provide an overview of ADHD psychoeducation needed to effectively conduct Session 1 of the MAPs for ADHD Program. This information is used to educate the participants new to or less familiar with the empirically based literature on ADHD and set the stage for effective mindful observing of ADHD-related behaviors and characteristics. The psychoeducation should build off of the MT's broader, up-to-date knowledge of the scientific literature on ADHD, either through reading the literature directly or through resources that summarize the literature (e.g., professional newsletters such as *The ADHD Report* or organizations such as the American Professional Society of ADHD and Related Disorders [*https://apsard.org*], the World Federation of ADHD [*www.adhd-federation.org*], the European Network Adult ADHD [*www.eunetworkadultadhd.com*], the Attention Deficit Disorder Association [*https://add.org*], the Canadian ADHD Resource Alliance [*www.caddra.ca*], and Children and Adults with Attention-Deficit/Hyperactivity Disorder [*https://chadd.org*]).

Overall, we encourage open dialogue in the group and discourage "lecturing" to participants. While we provide several topics, we don't expect that all of the content will be covered in full. The participants' questions and comments should guide the dialogue.

DIAGNOSTIC TERMINOLOGY

We often find that participants ask about the use of "ADD" versus "ADHD." It is helpful to explain to the group that ADD was the abbreviation used in DSM-III, but it was changed to ADHD in later editions. Typically, when participants use "ADD," it is a shorthand expression of "ADHD without hyperactivity" or "predominantly inattentive presentation." Some participants prefer the use of ADD because they assume ADHD implies that they have hyperactive-impulsive symptoms. In general, we provide the context for the diagnostic labels that we use, but ultimately find the language that the participant is comfortable with and build on that.

DIAGNOSTIC CRITERIA

We discuss DSM diagnostic criteria (American Psychiatric Association [APA], 2013) in MAPs, including the following criteria: symptom count, childhood onset, pervasiveness, functional impact, and the caution that symptoms should not be better accounted for by another mental disorder. We present the core nine inattentive symptoms and nine hyperactive-impulsive symptoms as they are listed in DSM-5 (APA, 2013)—please refer to the DSM-5 for the full list of 18 ADHD symptoms. However, instead of listing out the symptoms in a didactic fashion, we recommend first asking participants what they think of when they refer to ADHD. We then list on a whiteboard what the participants say, which typically includes the core symptoms. Once a list is complied, we help categorize the symptoms and also add symptoms that may not have been mentioned.

PERSISTENCE INTO ADULTHOOD

Historically ADHD was believed to be a childhood disorder that children simply outgrew. However, multiple longitudinal studies now demonstrate that this is not the case (Sibley, Mitchell, & Becker, 2016). Research shows that rates of ADHD persistence from childhood to adulthood depend on a number of factors, including symptom reporting source (e.g., self-report, parent report), symptom threshold levels, consideration of the functional impairment criterion, and study sample composition (e.g., early longitudinal studies were done predominantly with White males). Current best estimates of persistence are around 50%. In other words, about 50% of children with ADHD will continue to meet the diagnosis in the adulthood. Over the course of this discussion in MAPs, some participants may comment that they "didn't have ADHD as a child" or wonder why their ADHD wasn't "caught" as a child. Therefore, the MT needs to be prepared to discuss reasons for these perceptions (e.g., excessive parental and teacher assistance, high IQ helping to compensate for the symptoms, their symptoms were nondisruptive or not significantly impairing as a child, or their retrospective recall is not accurate).

PREVALENCE OF ADHD

The prevalence estimate of ADHD is around 5% of the adult population and is quite stable worldwide (Willcutt, 2012). To put that into perspective, the current adult population in the United States is about 245 million people (see *http://datacenter.kidscount.org*), which translates to over 12 million adults with ADHD living in the United States. Participants may be surprised to learn that despite common myths about pharmacological treatment for ADHD, most adults with ADHD are not currently prescribed medication for ADHD. For example, in one study, only 10.9% of adults with ADHD received treatment for ADHD in the previous 12 months (Kessler et al., 2006).

CAUSES OF ADHD

Causes of ADHD are not entirely known but include genetic and environmental etiologies. This is an extensive topic that is beyond the scope of this book, and for interested readers we recommend book-length discussions and reviews (e.g., Cortese, Faraone, & Sergeant, 2011; Nigg, 2006). For the purposes of this MAPs session, here are the important basic facts to cover:

- ADHD is considered a neurobiologically based disorder, meaning that having ADHD is often linked with differences in brain function and in physiological responding.
- ADHD is highly heritable (about 70%), but early environment factors such as maternal smoking during pregnancy, childhood lead exposure, and early developmental support are also linked to ADHD.
- Multiple genes are involved in ADHD, including dopaminergic genes. Therefore, genetics play a role, but it is likely many genes instead of a single gene.
- ADHD results in greater difficulty with self-regulation, including executive functioning (planning ahead, organization, and time management behaviors) and emotional regulation that are associated with frontal lobe functioning and subcortical areas.

One of the main points to convey to participants about the causes of ADHD is that there is still much we don't know about ADHD. Biology is certainly involved and plays a significant role, but it does not fully explain all cases of the disorder. Using metaphor for participants, the MT might state something like "just as there may be many paths up a mountain, there may be many paths to ADHD."

ADHD is a neurobiologically based condition that often continues into adulthood and can have different presentations.

NONDIAGNOSTIC CHARACTERISTICS OF ADHD

Inattention and hyperactivity-impulsivity are the primary symptom domains of ADHD, but for many adults with ADHD, these are not the main symptom domains reported. Difficulty with executive functions and regulating emotions is common in ADHD (Barkley & Murphy, 2010; Martel, 2009; Shaw et al., 2014). Problems with executive function include trouble with task initiation or completion, poor organization and planning, or difficulty with time management. Difficulties with emotion regulation might include becoming easily frustrated, difficulty recovering from feeling upset, and difficulty making sense out of what is going on emotionally "in the heat of the moment." Such emotional difficulties are a good target in ADHD treatments and appear to improve after mindfulness-based training (Mitchell et al., 2017) (see Chapter 2). Similarly, the tendency to act on "automatic pilot" or without awareness is common in ADHD and a direct target in mindfulness-based interventions (Mitchell et al., 2015). Rejection sensitivity has also been noted for those with ADHD. The MT can ask participants about these ADHD characteristics in their own life and keep their responses in mind when later discussing how mindfulness can help with ADHD.

HOW IS ADHD ASSESSED?

Presumably everyone in the group will have received a thorough, best-practice assessment of ADHD. However, we recommended asking participants about their opinions about this topic. The main point here is to emphasize that there is no definitive questionnaire or computer test for ADHD, nor are there any brain scan or genetic tests available to assess for ADHD. Instead, the "gold-standard" assessment in the ADHD field typically involves a thorough developmental assessment (e.g., prenatal history and childhood functioning at home, at school, and in social settings), use of standardized rating scales with multiple reporting sources, and a semistructured interview with an ADHD-informed clinician (Sibley et al., 2012).

REFRAMING COMMON ASSUMPTIONS ABOUT ADHD

Research studies comparing ADHD and non-ADHD samples have shown neurobiological differences, including differences in brain structure and activation. For example, studies using fMRI have identified dysfunctions in the lateral prefrontal cortex and its connections to the basal ganglia, as well as medial frontal, cingulate, and orbital frontal regions in ADHD samples (Rubia, Alegria, & Brinson, 2014). Differences are also expressed as overt behaviors others can observe (e.g., fidgeting) and covert behaviors others cannot observe (e.g., mind wandering) that create impairment. This association between neurobiological differences and behavior in a disorder that is pervasive across development is why we refer to ADHD as a neurodevelopmental disorder. However, the MT should consider how ADHD can also be framed in a hopeful way. For example, while reframing different kinds of psychiatric disorders as brain diseases tends to reduce blame toward individuals with the illness and self-blame, it also increases pessimism about prognosis of that disorder (Kvaale, Haslam, & Gottdiener, 2013; Lebowitz, Pyun, & Ahn, 2014; see Kichuk, Lebowitz, & Grover Adams, 2015, for a broader discussion on this topic). In contrast, ADHD symptoms can be conceptualized as normally distributed in the population (Frazier, Youngstrom, & Naugle, 2007; Levy et al., 1997), which might come as a surprise to participants who may have been thinking of ADHD as a purely binary construct (i.e., either you have it or you don't). Just like many other phenomena are normally distributed in the population—such as height, IQ, blood pressure, anxiety, and personality traits—so are ADHD symptoms. While discussing a medical/categorical model versus a dimensional model, the purpose is not to convince participants on how to view ADHD, but rather to expose them to a different way of thinking about ADHD. The dimensional model also shows the possibility that one can move along the continuum of symptom severity and that skill training or lifestyle change can help normalize the symptoms.

A common topic within the ADHD community is whether there are strengths associated with having ADHD or whether ADHD is a "gift." In addressing this controversial topic, the MT may ask participants to think about "adaptiveness" of behavior, pointing out that behavior occurs in the context of one's environment. For example, seminal research on childhood temperament by Thomas and Chess (1977) demonstrated how different traits or behaviors can be adaptive in different environments. While a certain behavior may be adaptive in one situation, it may not be adaptive in another. For ADHD, symptoms may be more apparent when there is a mismatch between a person's behavioral repertoire and the demands of his or her environment (Jensen et al., 1997). This is not to say that ADHD is a culturally bound disorder (worldwide prevalence is actually quite high, e.g., Willcutt, 2012), but instead that the MT wants participants to not simply see their behavior as "good" or "bad," but as skillful or adaptive. One way to think about "adaptiveness" is to ask if a person's ADHD-related behaviors are in the service of larger concrete goals or broader values. If "yes," then that's an indication they're on the right track; if "no," then maybe they are not.

The MT can also help participants conceptualize their own unique strengths in the context of treatment. Although ADHD in adulthood is associated with a number of maladaptive outcomes (Hechtman et al., 2016), everybody has strengths. For example, adults with ADHD may seek out professions or outlets in which typical characteristics associated with ADHD are more adaptive (White & Shah, 2011). An adversity may also help develop certain strengths, such as persistence and excelling in a sport to counter ADHD-related difficulties (e.g., the U.S. Olympic swimmer Michael Phelps is said to have used swimming as an outlet for his ADHD when he was a child). The MT can remind participants that it is important to think about their own strengths and how they can use them in working on the difficulties they face.

Finally, the MT can discuss how ADHD is somewhat of a misnomer: it is not a complete deficit or inability to pay attention, but rather it is an issue with *paying attention to the right thing at the right time*. More accurately, ADHD is a difficulty in attention regulation. Hyperfocus can also happen in ADHD and may be both adaptive (e.g., intense productive time) or maladaptive (e.g., losing track of time). Accordingly, mindfulness involves "paying attention to attention" and is a way to strengthen one's ability to regulate attention. When the mind wanders off, participants can use mindfulness to pause and "catch their minds wandering," let go of negatively judging themselves for this behavior, and redirect their attention back to the intended focus. Mindfulness practice emphasizes this nonjudgmental, curious, and compassionate observation, thereby letting go of frustration, shame, and a whole host of other negative emotions that accompany self-criticism. Overall, mindfulness involves both focusing and monitoring of attention, which are practices that strengthen self-regulation in ADHD.

PART II

MAPs FOR ADHD PROGRAM

Seeing the Forest for the Trees

Before the MT dives into the program, we want to make sure that we clearly convey the "structural bones" of MAPs that guide the selection of mindfulness practice for each session. The structure creates a gradual introduction of mindfulness practice, starting with single-focus and attention-monitoring training designed to move away from the "automatic pilot" mode (Sessions 1–3) and later intentionally applying the skills to experience and self-regulate inner experiences of body sensations, thoughts, emotions, interactions, or awareness itself (Sessions 4–8). The structure guides selection of the current mindfulness practices in MAPs, but it can also invite new practices, as long as they address each session's intention as to what is being trained. Once this guiding structure is clearly understood, MTs can use their knowledge and creativity to introduce new mindfulness practices. Such flexibility is especially useful when working in individual therapy or when modifying the length or duration of the group training.

Sessions 1–3 Intention Moving Away from Automatic Pilot Mode; Strengthening Control and Monitoring of Attention	
Session Theme	Core Mindful Awareness Practices
1. Introduction to ADHD and Mindfulness: Reframing of ADHD	Playing with Attention and Five Senses Mindful Eating Mindfulness of Breath
2. Mindful Awareness of ADHD Patterns: "What Is My ADHD Like?"	Mindfulness of Breath
3. Mindful Awareness of Sound, Breath, and Body	Mindfulness of Sound, Breath, and Body Mindful Movement Mindful Walking S.T.O.P.
Sessions 4–8 Intention **New Relationship to the Inner Experiences; Deepening Awareness and Ability to Choose Responses (Self-Regulation)**	
Session Theme	Core Mindful Awareness Practices
4. Mindful Awareness of Body Sensations	Body Scan Working with Discomfort
5. Mindful Awareness of Thoughts	Mindfulness of Thoughts (Mind Like a Sky)
6. Mindful Awareness of Emotions	R.A.I.N. Loving-Kindness
7. Mindful Awareness of Presence and Interactions	Mindful Presence Mindful Listening and Speaking
8. Mindful Awareness as a Life Journey	Mindful Presence Mindful Walking

SESSION 1

Introduction to ADHD and Mindfulness

Reframing of ADHD

SESSION SUMMARY

Overview

The program begins with a session devoted to participant and MT introductions, ADHD overview, basic information about mindfulness practice, and the first experiential exercises.

Session Outline

1) Getting started[1]
2) Welcome and introductions
   - General orientation to a group setting and rules of confidentiality
   - "Getting to Know You" activity
   - Short reflection on motivation to be in the class
   - Group structure and format overview
3) ADHD introduction
   - Sharing about living with ADHD
   - ADHD psychoeducation and reframing assumptions about ADHD
4) Break

[1]This part of the session outline is not included in the participant handout because it involves considerations for the MT prior to the start of the session.

5) Mindfulness introduction
    - Definition of mindfulness and how it can help manage ADHD
    - Treatment outcome research on ADHD and mindfulness
    - Introduction to attention and the five senses: Playing with Visual Attention and Awareness (*Exercise 1.1*) and Mindful Eating (*Exercise 1.2*)
    - Sitting meditation introduction and Mindfulness of Breath (5 minutes) (*Exercise 1.3*)
6) Closing
    - Discussion of home practice

Home Practice

1) Formal mindfulness practice: Mindfulness of Breath (5 minutes per day)
2) Informal mindfulness practice:
    - Mindfulness of a routine daily activity, such as eating, showering, or brushing teeth
    - Brief mindful check-ins: "telephone breath" or "red light breath"

GETTING STARTED

The overarching goals of this session are twofold.

The *first goal* of this session is to establish a cohesive atmosphere following standard group therapy guidelines. As in group therapy in general, a supportive group dynamic is central to participants disclosing their experiences to others in the group. The MT will discuss guidelines for participation so that the group encourages a respectful attitude toward others and emphasis on sharing of inner experience (versus commenting on others' experience).

The *second goal* is to give the participants an overview of this treatment, including what ADHD is and how mindfulness training can be helpful in this condition. Although this introduction is led by the MT and there are particular areas that need to be addressed, the process of teaching is collaborative. The initial didactic format should quickly transition to a discussion with participants that allows for addressing questions and assumptions. The MT can also use a board to write down answers from the group as a way to engage participants and facilitate the discussion. Since mindfulness practices are best learned experientially, in addition to a discussion of what mindfulness meditation is, this session introduces simple guided meditations.

Also, before getting started, the MT should consider administering measures to track treatment progress (see Chapter 3 for examples) and determine how often these measures should be completed. Although ADHD symptoms will be a typical target (e.g., the severity of the 18 DSM symptoms), other potential treatment targets can be considered: poor executive functioning, emotion dysregulation, or perception of stress, for example.

WELCOME AND INTRODUCTIONS

General Orientation to a Group Setting and Rules of Confidentiality

After a brief introduction of the trainers (full introductions are provided later), the MT sets the context for the group as a nonjudgmental setting in which participants can feel comfortable sharing their present-moment experiences. Some participants may be familiar with a psychotherapy group format, while others may be new to group therapy altogether. We also find that some participants have previously participated in other mindfulness programs, while some are novices to meditation. Because of such variability and assumptions of what group therapy is in general, it is important to cover some basic information about the MAPs for ADHD Program.

Confidentiality and Sharing in the Group

These are important topics to discuss in order to establish the group as a setting that is nurturing. Typical confidentiality guidelines involve agreeing to not discuss other people or their stories outside of the group. In MAPs, it is also suggested that "others sharing serves as a mirror to reflect on ourselves." Therefore, even in group, rather than participants providing advice to others, they are encouraged to reflect on and discuss only their own experiences. For this group rule and any others, the MT should list them on a board or display them in some way over the course of the discussion. Participants can also write out the notes using Handout 1.1.

Support Outside of the Group

An option for creating support outside of the group is the use of an individual "mindfulness buddy." This is similar to having an "exercise buddy" to keep one motivated for physical exercise. This support strategy has been utilized in a child and adolescent ADHD mindfulness program and found helpful (Bögels & Restifo, 2014). Participants can form a dyad and text each other once per day to prompt an awareness of breath at that moment. Additional social support strategies might involve having regular discussions about experiences with mindfulness exercises, sharing mindfulness readings, or practicing formal mindfulness exercises together outside of the weekly group trainings. Other options for a "mindfulness buddy" could involve friends or family members outside the program, or seeking support elsewhere in the community (e.g., online communities that promote mindfulness meditation training).

Verbal Impulsivity

Different aspects of verbal impulsivity among participants is another topic that frequently emerges. Participants are invited to nonjudgmentally notice a common tendency to interrupt or talk too much in a group and to practice self-correcting such behavior. It's important to ask participants to focus on self-awareness and self-correcting versus correcting other members of the group. The MT should also let participants know ahead of time that sometimes it will be necessary for the MT to redirect the discussion to remedy this common issue for adults diagnosed with ADHD. Again, the MT should emphasize that such redirecting is meant to foster nonjudgmental self-awareness and self-regulation, and hopefully will not be experienced as criticism or shaming. For example, the MT can say to the participants, "I will use the meditation bell as a gentle reminder to wrap up comments as a way to manage the common ADHD pitfall of talking too much or interrupting." Or the MT can use certain nonjudgmental phrases that encourage collaboration between the MT and the participant in curbing the excessive talking, such as "I'm noticing that we have only a few minutes before we move on to the next topic. I want to both understand what you're telling us and also make sure that we get to the next topic in the next few minutes. Can you help me with this?" For interrupting, an example of something the MT might say is "I just noticed that Bill was saying something about having trouble practicing a formal mindfulness exercise in the mornings, but that we didn't hear the end of the difficulty he's having." This introduction to in-session behaviors helps the MT manage the group and "set the stage" to facilitate discussions about ADHD behaviors in a future session in a compassionate and nonthreatening way. This also starts setting a tone for mindful listening and speaking.

Lateness

This is another potentially disruptive in-session behavior that regularly arises in ADHD groups. After all, ADHD is a disorder characterized by difficulty with time management. Late arrivals can be disruptive, especially during a formal meditation exercise, and should be addressed proactively (e.g., the MT can put a sign on the door to wait until the exercise is finished). The MT should also discuss with the group that adults with ADHD tend to underestimate the amount of time required for tasks, transitions, or travel, and offer solutions, such as setting a realistic time to leave home instead of rushing at the last minute. The MT can suggest that participants "approximate up" by adding 20–30% more time (e.g., if they say they can drive to the clinic in 15 minutes, the estimate should be at least 20 minutes). The MT might ask participants to consider how long it takes them to drive from their point of origin to wherever the group is held, how long it takes to park, how long it takes to walk from the parking spot to the building, and how long it takes to check in. Uncontrollable variables such as heavy traffic or a long line at the front desk to check in should be considered as well.

Forgetfulness, Inattention, and Impatience

These behaviors are other common ADHD behaviors that may impact participation in the program. For example, the participants may forget group materials, "zone out" and miss parts of group discussions, and get impatient if the pace of the group appears to be too slow. Similar to handling verbal behavior or lateness in session, the MT can discuss the importance of nonjudgmentally observing the behavior as an initial step to problem solving how to handle it in the group.

Reluctance to Share in the Group

Reluctance toward sharing can arise for some participants and the MT should address this common difficulty. The MT can offer compassionate encouragement and acceptance that speaking in a group often creates some discomfort and that such discomfort can be noted mindfully. At the same time, to encourage the participants who may be shy to share in the group, the MT can point out that "our sharing is a gift for each other." It can also be helpful to emphasize that "there is no right or wrong way to experience mindfulness training. It is important that each one of you brings curiosity to how your experience unfolds and any reaction that comes up can be looked at together in the group."

ADAPTATION TO INDIVIDUAL THERAPY

While some of the confidentially rules (e.g., talking to others outside of group or commenting on others' behavior) are not relevant to the patient in individual therapy, the MT should discuss any relevant disruptive in-session behaviors, such as lateness or excessive talking. As in the group context, through modeling, the goal is to build the patient's own nonjudgmental self-awareness and capacity for self-correction.

"Getting to Know You" Activity

After the initial group guidelines are discussed, the MT leads an activity that introduces participants to each other. All participants and the MT meet in a circle and the MT introduces him- or herself. Whereas earlier the brief MT introduction entailed providing a name and title (e.g., psychologist, psychiatrist, clinical social worker), now the MT may want to disclose how they became interested in mindfulness meditation practice or a little bit about their own personal practice of mindfulness. The MT asks each participant to introduce him- or herself as an "ice breaker" (allow about 5 minutes per person). Here are examples of prompting ice breakers:

- "Please briefly introduce yourself and tell us something interesting about you, like a hobby that you enjoy."
- "Please briefly introduce yourself and tell us something that is unique about you."
- "Please briefly introduce yourself and tell us about a strength of yours."

Short Reflection on Motivation to Be in the Class

After the brief ice breaker above, the MT invites participants to reflect on the questions related to each person's motivation for being in the mindfulness training (allow about 5 minutes per person). If the group is large, sharing can be done in dyads first, then asking a few volunteers to share in the group. Sample prompts to initiate discussion include:

- "What brings you here?"
- "What motivated you to join this class?"
- "What would you like to learn from this class?"
- "On your way to group today, what was one thing that you looked forward to and one thing that you were concerned about?"

Of note, it is not uncommon that some participants might have enrolled in the group in response to requests from family members who are frustrated with their behavior. Such members may not be fully committed to attending the group (i.e., they're attending to get someone "off their back," not to learn how to cope with ADHD behaviors). This above brief motivational exercise may help the ambivalent participant identify or affirm motivations to attend the training with full engagement.

ADAPTATION TO INDIVIDUAL THERAPY

The reflection on motivation can be explored more deeply in individual therapy. The MT may make efficient use of this opportunity by examining the pros and cons of initiating treatment (short term and long term) to help patients appreciate the challenges they may encounter over the course of treatment. Also, this discussion may lead to more individualized treatment goals than what can be covered in a group setting. Similar to strategies found in CBT for adult ADHD, the MT can help patients identify how controllable these goals are and help start tailoring future sessions.

Group Structure and Format Overview

The MT discusses meeting dates and times, but keeps logistics of the group to a minimum since they are reiterated in the handout with group rules (Handout 1.1).

The general structure of sessions is reviewed, including that each session starts and ends with a formal mindfulness meditation. Differences between this type of group and other types of group therapies are also discussed. For instance, discussion in this group typically focuses on present experiences and how to translate insights learned from mindfulness practice into daily life with ADHD. This also means that the MT will have to redirect participants at times when the topic of conversation drifts. It is the MTs task to strike a balance between allowing for support offered by the group discussion with maintaining an emphasis on the session's agenda and experiential mindfulness practice.

Although it will be reviewed toward the conclusion of the session, it is worthwhile here to briefly comment on the importance of attendance and home practice. For example, the MT might state that "practicing mindfulness is mental training that, like physical training, needs repeated practice." The analogy of "attention muscle" that gets stronger every time a person engages in mindful noting can be used. The MT should also request to be informed in the event of an absence. In the event of an absence, the MT will want participants to consider how they can "catch up" on what they missed. Regarding adherence to home practices, the MT should ask participants about typical barriers to adopting new behaviors, and offer solutions. To help with forgetfulness of appointments, the MT can send an email the day before a session or help participants set reminders on their phones. The MT can also send a "summary email" at the end of each group session, reminding them of exercises in between sessions (see the end of this chapter for an example email). Overall, the message is that regular attendance to the group, formal meditation, and informal (in daily life) mindfulness practice are central to gaining the benefits of this group.

When communicating instructions, the MT should embrace guidelines used in teaching children with ADHD, including giving brief requests with clear step-by-step directions. Executive function deficits are common in both children and adults with ADHD and "short and to-the-point" communication is often most effective.

> **ADAPTATION TO INDIVIDUAL THERAPY**
>
> As opposed to a summary email that the MT sends to participants in a group, in individual therapy the MT may encourage patients to list the home practice for the week in the session and then review the list together. The MT can provide specific feedback to ensure that patients understand the tasks and help set up reminders for practice.

ADHD INTRODUCTION

Sharing about Living with ADHD

Although the MT may want to provide a didactic lecture on ADHD, we find that participants' sharing about their experience of living with ADHD is a better, more engaging way to start the discussion. The following questions are asked to prompt the discussion:

- "What is ADHD?"
- "How is ADHD affecting your life?" or "What effect does ADHD have on your life?"
- "Tell me about your daily experience with ADHD."
- "What has been helpful in managing challenges you've faced because of ADHD?"
- "What do you 'like' and 'dislike' about your ADHD?"

The MT can use a board to write down key words expressed by the participants, which can facilitate the psychoeducation points below.

ADHD Psychoeducation and Reframing Assumptions about ADHD

The MT uses the participants' own comments about their ADHD as a springboard for more formal didactic information about ADHD. The MT can also pose questions to participants to direct them to important topics—for example, "When do you think was the earliest reference to ADHD in the medical literature?"; participants might be surprised that learn that that answer is 1775 (Barkley & Peters, 2012). Below are some areas that MTs will want to cover, although it is important for MTs to have a working knowledge of the ADHD literature so that they are not solely relying on the points below.

Diagnostic Criteria for ADHD

Prior to enrolling in the MAPs Program, participants should have received a diagnosis of ADHD and presumably the diagnostic criteria to make that diagnosis was described at that time. However, participants may have forgotten the information, been misinformed, or it was inadequately described. In any case, we find it helpful to walk through the DSM-5 criteria. The key points include:

- There are 18 symptoms composed of two symptom clusters: inattentive symptoms (composed of nine items) and hyperactive-impulsive symptoms (composed of nine items). At least five of either inattentive or hyperactive-impulsive symptoms have to be endorsed as occurring "often" or "very often."
- In addition, ADHD symptoms require an age of onset during childhood (i.e., by age 12).
- Further, symptoms must be pervasive across settings and functionally impairing, and cannot be better accounted for by another disorder.
- Based on the symptom presentation, DSM-5 describes different presentation styles: combined presentation, predominantly inattentive presentation, and predominantly hyperactive-impulsive presentation.
- The severity level can be specified as mild, moderate, or severe. In addition, for cases that have not met the full criteria for the past 6 months but symptoms still result in functional impairment, the "in partial remission" specifier is an option.

Additional topics include diagnostic terminology ("Is it ADD or ADHD?"), persistence into adulthood, prevalence and causes of ADHD, associated characteristics (executive function difficulties, emotional regulation problems, low self-esteem), and "gold-standard" assessment. Other common assumptions or questions (e.g., "Is ADHD a disorder or simply a brain difference?" and "Are there strengths that come with ADHD?") can be elaborated on, especially as prompted by participants' sharing. See Chapter 4 for an in-depth discussion of how we address such topics in the group.

BREAK

This is approximately the midpoint in the session, where a 5- to 10-minute break is taken.

MINDFULNESS INTRODUCTION

Definition of Mindfulness and How It Can Help Manage ADHD

"What is mindfulness and how can it help manage your ADHD?" The MT poses this question to the group and elicits examples from participants to guide the conversation. Mindfulness is defined in many ways. This is a complicated and nuanced topic (Grossman, 2008, 2011; Kang & Whittingham, 2010) and the MT may have their own favorite way of defining the concept. In our groups we offer the "classic" definition of "mindfulness means paying attention in a particular way: on purpose, in the present moment, and nonjudgmentally" (Kabat-Zinn, 1990) and show how there are two key steps: attention and attitude. The attention step involves bringing attention to an aspect of the present-moment experience (e.g., breath, sound, or thinking) and the attitude step involves adapting a nonjudgmental, curious, open, accepting, or compassionate stance. Another helpful way to define mindfulness is via the Five Facet Mindfulness Questionnaire, which includes five trait-like skills: observing, describing, acting with awareness, nonjudging of inner experience, and nonreactivity to inner experience (Baer et al., 2008). For participants who are inclined to do so, invite them to take notes on Handout 1.2 during this discussion.

In discussing mindfulness, we also review the current neuroscience findings, highlighting the potential of meditation training to improve self-regulation and modify brain functioning over time via neuroplasticity. For example, we describe one recent study demonstrating that mindfulness meditation training functionally couples the default mode network with a region important to executive control (Creswell et al., 2016)—as we reviewed in Part I, these are areas associated with ADHD as well. The mechanism of neuroplasticity is highlighted (e.g., MTs can say, "Neuroplasticity or brain changes happen when you are paying attention on purpose while repeating an experience") and correlated with the ongoing mindfulness practice. Brain studies by Merzenich and colleagues (Merzenich, Nahum, & Van Vleet, 2013; Merzenich, Van Vleet, & Nahum, 2014) or brain studies of piano or violin players can be mentioned to demonstrate how repeated practice is needed to acquire a new skill and engender associated brain changes (e.g., it takes 1,200 hours to learn to play a violin; Strayhorn, 2002).

To fully learn about mindfulness, one must experience the actual practice of it. Such experiential learning can be contrasted with didactic learning or learning about something new by talking about it. The MT explains how, in this group, both forms of learning are important. The MT—especially those who are used to an active, didactic role with patients—should be cautious about getting caught up in too much discussion about mindfulness to the point that the actual formal practice of mindfulness is shortchanged and experiential learning is limited.

Common misconceptions of meditation practice should be addressed by the MT, such as "Do I need to empty my mind?" or "Do I have to sit in a special way for the meditation to be effective?" The MT should normalize common difficulties of meditating such as mind wandering or restlessness. These can be especially pronounced for adults with ADHD, yet mindfulness practice can still proceed and be effective. The MT should instruct participants on the importance of becoming aware of their own moment-to-moment experience and that how they respond to themselves (i.e., with curiosity and compassion) is more important than achieving steady concentration or complete calmness in the body. The MT should also discuss how mindfulness is different from relaxation: while quiet relaxation is encouraged in mindfulness practice, mindful observation can be applied to any mind-body state, including moments of tension, moments of noise, in the midst of an activity, and during movement.

The concept of being stuck in "automatic pilot" is introduced with examples of how we can all become unaware and act out of habit. The MT describes how being on automatic pilot can lead to getting stuck in a problem without considering all available options (i.e., a more helpful/adaptive/skillful behavior). The MT can use discussion points from the section above on "characteristics of ADHD" here. For example, the MT may ask participants something like "Have you ever blindly reacted to a thought or a feeling on 'automatic pilot' and dropped a more important task for a less important one, only to later on think to yourself 'that wasn't a good decision'?" The MT can direct participants to Handout 1.3 to think about how being on automatic pilot unfolds in their own experience.

Treatment Outcome Research on ADHD and Mindfulness

As a last point, we briefly review the treatment outcome literature for mindfulness-based interventions for ADHD (see Chapter 2). We touch on the rationale for using mindfulness in ADHD (based on findings in non-ADHD samples), how many studies have been conducted with ADHD adults, what is known about mindfulness's impact on core ADHD symptoms and functional impairment, and what are the current gaps in our scientific knowledge. The main points of discussion are:

- Mindfulness has been shown to improve aspects of attentional functioning, which is a core difficulty in ADHD.
- Mindfulness has been shown to improve impulsive responding, which is a core difficulty with ADHD.
- Mindfulness has been shown to help people regulate their mood when upset, which is a common difficulty that people with ADHD face.

ADAPTATION TO INDIVIDUAL THERAPY

The introductory sections on ADHD and mindfulness can be covered in a similar discussion format in an individual therapy setting. As in a group format, the MT should be aware of balancing the need to be comprehensive with the time needed to complete the full session agenda. Given the shorter duration of individual therapy sessions, it may be around this point that the MT may conclude and wait to resume the remainder of the content the following week. In that case, we would recommend that patients leave the session having received some experiential practice with formal mindfulness meditation. You may decide to introduce and practice the 5-minute Mindfulness of Breath exercise (*Exercise 1.3*).

The exercises that follow this box—*Exercises 1.1, 1.2,* and *1.3*—do not require much adaptation in individual therapy.

Introduction to Attention and the Five Senses

Difficulty with attention is a prominent feature of ADHD. To engender curious observation of attention, the MT should ask participants what they think attention is and how it differs across different situations. It is helpful to introduce a scientific model of attention. While there are different ways to describe attentional functioning, we use the attention network model developed by Michael Posner (Posner et al., 2006). This model describes attention to be composed of three main networks: alerting, orienting, and conflict detection (also called executive attention). Here are brief definitions of each:

- *Alerting* has to do with readying or gearing up attention to respond to experiences and involves maintaining good alertness over time (i.e., think "vigilance" and "alert arousal").
- *Orienting* has to do with movement of attention toward a sensory stimulus or shifting attention from one thing to another (i.e., think about reading as you read from one side of the page to the other).
- *Conflict detection* has to do with choosing a controlling response and is involved

with paying attention despite distractions (i.e., think about reading a book and your computer alerting you that you received a new email with a sound—you're engaging conflict detection when you hear that sound and continue reading).

The MT can use a flashlight analogy to further explain the concept of attention:

- *Alerting* is like turning on the flashlight.
- *Orienting* is like pointing it toward what you want to see.
- *Conflict detection* is keeping the light in one place even if something distracting occurs.
- Also, like a flashlight, wherever you place your attention, the spot becomes illuminated and more clearly perceived.

The MT can ask participants which of these attention networks seem to be most applicable to them in day-to-day life.

PLAYING WITH VISUAL ATTENTION AND AWARENESS (EXERCISE 1.1)

Using a famous visual illusion called Rubin's vase (Figure S1.1), this exercise demonstrates the interplay of paying attention and being aware.

To facilitate the observation, the MT asks participants:

- "What do you see when you look at this picture?"
- "A vase?"
- "How about two faces?"
- "How about both the vase and the faces simultaneously?"

The MT discusses with participants that the key here is that awareness changes depending on placement of our attention.

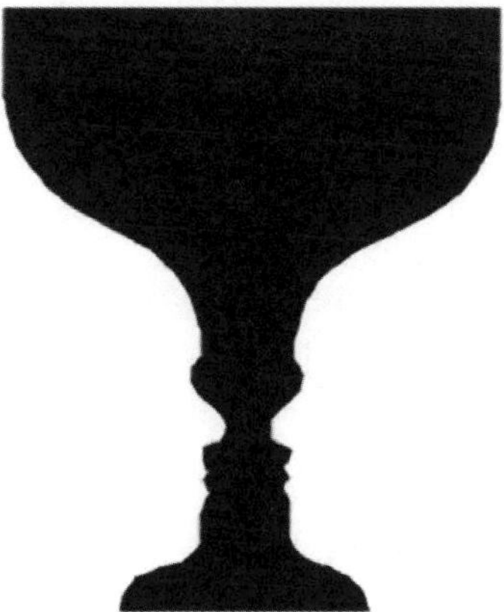

FIGURE S1.1. Rubin's vase.

After this exercise, the MT invites participants to share their experiences with this experiential practice. The MT models curiosity, openness, willingness to experience something new, and being nonjudgmental. Example prompts include:

- "How was your experience with this exercise?"
- "Did you find it easy or difficult?"
- "How do you think this exercise relates to your ADHD?"

MINDFUL EATING (EXERCISE 1.2)

The purpose of this exercise is to purposefully bring attention/awareness to the five senses and notice how the change alters the quality of moment-by-moment experience of eating. This is modeled after the "Eating a Raisin" exercise used in MBSR training (see Kabat-Zinn, 1990). A raisin or other food (e.g., grapes, chocolates, or any other food options that may be of more interest to the group) can be used to conduct the exercise. Here's a script of what the MT might say when leading the exercise:

> Now we are going to practice awareness of all five senses using food. I am going to pass around these raisins. Please take one and put it in your hand—don't eat it yet. [*Make sure each participant receives a raisin.*]
>
> Look at the raisin in your hand. Think about where it came from. See if you can imagine how it got to you. There was someone who planted grapevines, there was the soil and the rain and the sun. There were people who tended it, and when it was a grape, someone picked it and dried it. It was probably put in a truck and driven to the grocery store, maybe it came on an airplane. Now think about the whole story of this raisin. Imagine all the things that made this raisin come to be here in your hand. [*Pause 30 seconds to allow participants to reflect in silence.*]
>
> Now look more closely at your raisin. Imagine that you just dropped from Mars and have never seen such a thing as this object in your hand. Bring curiosity to it and first inspect it, noticing the texture, the color of the raisin or anything else that may be there. Inspect it visually and notice its texture, color, and shape. Examine the highlights where the light shines . . . the darker hollows and folds of it. Let your eyes explore every part of it as if you had never seen such a thing before.
>
> Next, touch it with your finger. Roll it and feel any texture or sensation, such as stickiness or dryness.
>
> Now holding your raisin up, bring it to your ear, paying attention to how you move your arm, and your hand and your elbow to bring the raisin to your ear. See if you hear any sounds that may be there or perhaps you notice the *absence* of sound. When you roll it between your fingers, ask yourself if you hear anything.
>
> Next, bringing it slowly to your nose, smell the raisin and notice its scent. Notice if you feel hungry. Notice if it feels like you want to eat the raisin.
>
> Now very slowly bring your hand to your mouth, but don't put the raisin in your mouth yet. Maybe you'll notice your hand and arm know exactly where to put it, perhaps noticing your mouth watering as it comes up. Close your eyes. Feel the raisin touching your lips and observe any sensations that may be there, for example feeling coldness or roughness.

And if, when you are doing this, any thoughts come to mind about "What a strange thing we are doing" or "What is the point of this?" or "I don't like these," then just notice them as thoughts and bring your awareness back to the object.

When you are ready, with your eyes closed, next place the raisin in your mouth. Become aware of how it feels to have the raisin in your mouth. You may observe your tongue movement, the saliva, and the chewing of your teeth. [*Pause.*] Now very consciously take a bite into it and notice the taste it releases. You may notice if you chew on the right side of your mouth or the left side. Or, notice if you can smell the raisin while you are chewing it. Notice if the raisin is changing its shape or taste while you chew it, notice the saliva in your mouth and the change in consistency of this object. Notice any sounds associated with chewing. Be curious about your own experience, whatever it is.

Then, when you feel ready to swallow, see if you can first detect the intention to swallow as it comes up, so that even this is experienced consciously before you actually swallow it. [*Pause.*] Finally notice the act of swallowing, noting that your body is now one raisin heavier than before.

Now I am going to ring the bell to end the meditation. Listen to the whole sound of the bell, and when you cannot hear the sound of the bell anymore, open your eyes. [*Ring bell.*]

The MT asks questions to facilitate the discussion and looks for opportunities to link mindful eating practice to ADHD patterns.

Question Examples

- "How was your experience with this exercise?"
- "What did you notice about the raisin that you don't typically notice?"
- "How do you think this exercise relates to your ADHD?"

The MT encourages participants to be curious about their reactions and let go of judging them as "good" or "bad." If negative emotions come up during the exercise (e.g., frustration, impatience, restlessness), the MT suggests participants explore them more deeply by asking how they manifest in their body, thoughts, or other emotions. Participants are invited to notice these emotions with compassion and continue to observe them with curiosity.

The MT also looks for opportunities to tie participants' experiences to ADHD. For example, the MT can suggest that noticing urges/desires (i.e., the urge to eat the raisin right away) or aversion (i.e., not wanting to taste the raisin) paves a way for noticing ADHD patterns such as "noticing the feeling you get just before you 'put something off' or the feeling right before saying something that you later regret"). The MT can also explain how feelings of boredom or craving for novelty are common in ADHD. The MT can elaborate that turning to the five senses is one way to change participants' experience with something that is important to them but might elicit boredom (e.g., needing to clean the dishes in the kitchen yet telling oneself "I'll do it later" and procrastinating). With mindful observing, even mundane activities can feel new and exciting, such as something we do every day: eating. By using the five senses, an everyday experience might change and it can feel like something never done before.

Sitting Meditation Introduction and Mindfulness of Breath

Review of Posture, Using a Meditation Pillow or Chair

The MT discusses sitting meditation posture (i.e., an upright, posture of dignity) and the use of a chair, meditation pillow, or other tools used with sitting meditation (blankets, meditation benches) for a formal sitting meditation exercise. The goal is to familiarize and demystify meditation accessories and the rules for meditation.

MINDFULNESS OF BREATH (5 MINUTES) (EXERCISE 1.3)

Instructions are given for basic breath awareness exercise. Participants are taught to settle their attention in the field of bodily sensations, attending particularly to the sensations associated with the breath. The nose, the chest, and the abdomen are given as the three places one can pay attention to breathing. After exploring each site, participants are invited to pick one spot and notice the sensations associated with each in-breath and each out-breath. While maintaining mindfulness of breathing, they cultivate introspective alertness of their mental states, noting in particular what happens to their attention (i.e., focused vs. distracted). When distracted, participants are taught to return to their breath as the anchor for their attention. The alternative of putting one's hand on one's chest or abdomen and noting its movement is given as another way to observe breathing. Here's a script of how you might lead the group through this exercise:

[*Ring bell.*]

In this exercise, you'll focus and monitor your attention to the sensation of your breath.

In the process you will also learn to catch yourself when distracted.

Find a relaxed and comfortable sitting position. Keep your back straight and relaxed as if you are sitting in a posture of dignity. Place your hands on your lap or beside you.

Close your eyes or keep them half closed and resting in one spot.

Set an intention to practice focusing and staying with your breath for the next few minutes.

Take a deep breath and allow yourself to simply rest in the present moment.

Let your usual preoccupations or need to do something else fall into the background.

Focus on your breath in one spot: your nostrils, chest, belly.

Bring in your full attention and notice the natural flow of air coming in . . . and going out . . . notice the natural rhythm of this breath and take a moment to notice this rhythm that has been going on all day . . . the only difference between your breath now and then is that you are more aware of it.

Keep the focus on your breathing, "being with" each in-breath for its full duration, then each out-breath for its full duration as if you are riding the wave of your breathing.

We will practice this in silence for a few minutes. Remember, if your mind wanders off 100 times, gently bring it back 100 times. [*Pause.*]

Where is your attention right now? If you notice that your mind has wandered off, such as to sounds outside or to your thoughts, that's okay; simply and gently remind yourself of your intention and return to the breath. Practice being kind to yourself. Don't judge your experience as good or bad. Simply notice the experience of how your mind works and allow yourself to come back to your breath.

As we end this meditation, offer yourself some appreciation for taking the time to pause, for training your attention and awareness, and for connecting more fully with yourself in the present moment.

[*Ring bell.*]

As will be typical after each experiential exercise, the MT discusses the practice with the participants. Here, the MT can point out how a basic breath exercise can help with stress, awareness and attention, and emotion regulation.

Question Examples to Initiate Discussion

- "How was your experience with this exercise?"
- "What did you notice about the breath that you don't typically notice?"
- "How do you think this exercise relates to your ADHD?"

CLOSING

Discussion of Home Practice

The MT goes through instructions on setting up a time and a place for sitting practice (i.e., ask each participant, "Where and when will you practice?," then "List it on your sheet") (see Handout 1.4). It is helpful to anticipate challenges people with ADHD may face as they set goals to practice mindfulness for the week and how to overcome them. For example, participants may want to use visual reminders, alarms, or ask a mindfulness buddy to text them. It may be helpful to practice at consistent times of the day, such as while waiting for their coffee to brew or while waiting for the computer to turn on.

The MT discusses the difference between formal and informal home practice. The following are the basic points to convey (also summarized in Handout 1.4).

The 5-minute Mindfulness of Breath exercise each day with recorded guidance is the formal practice. For this practice and all other formal meditation practices in MAPs, MTs can refer participants to the downloadable resources on The Guilford Press website (see the box at the end of the table of contents).

There are two informal practice suggestions for this week.

1. Noticing the five senses in daily life, such as being in nature and noticing sounds, colors, shapes, textures, and scents around you. Other examples can include mindfulness of a routine daily activity: eating, showering, or brushing teeth.
   - *Eating.* Tune in to the sensory input for a few minutes each day. This should be similar to the raisin exercise.
   - *Showering.* Notice the coolness or warmth of the water. How do you start? Shampoo first? Work from the top to bottom? Bottom to top? Be in the moment when you shower and be an observer of what you might otherwise do by habit and while on automatic pilot.
2. "Telephone breath" (taking a mindful breath every time the phone rings) is suggested for awareness of breath in daily life. Similarly, participants can practice

a "red light breath," which involves intentionally taking a mindful breath after stopping at a red light (after they've come to a complete stop and remind them to keep their eyes open if they are driving). Further, the MT can ask participants to practice these exercises (and the other informal exercises listed above) as soon as they can—perhaps even do something right after group like make their phone ring just for the sake of practicing these applications of mindfulness as soon as possible and therefore establish a foundation of adherence to at-home work for the group.

The Weekly Home Practice Sheet (Handout 1.4) is given at the end of session. The handout includes the formal and informal mindfulness suggestions. Participants can write down the formal and informal practices and any other notes they want. The MT asks participants to recall why they are in the group and to adopt a curious attitude toward mindfulness and immerse themselves to "give it a fair shot." The MT can use a metaphor to illustrate this point, such as "It's the difference between standing at the edge of the pool debating whether you'll enjoy swimming versus just jumping in and swimming—you'll get more from this group when you 'jump in' and practice formal and informal exercises."

If the MT decides to send a summary email to help participants recall session content and tasks to complete at home prior to the next session, here's an example:

It was great to meet most of you last night at our first group meeting!

Here's what we went over:

- Group Rules overview
- Introductions
- ADHD overview
- Mindful Eating
- Mindfulness and ADHD
- Mindfulness of Breath: Exercise and discussion

Here's what we went over for home practice this week (please do your best to record using the log provided in your binder):

1. Daily formal mindfulness practice. A link to recorded guided meditations is available on The Guilford Press website (see the box at the end of the table of contents).
2. Daily informal mindfulness practice to enhance awareness of the five senses
3. Daily informal mindfulness practice: mindful check-in

My office number is [*enter your phone number*] and my email address is [*enter your email address*]. If you anticipate you'll be late next session or have a planned absence, please let me know if you haven't already. I look forward to seeing everyone next week!

SESSION 2

Mindful Awareness of ADHD Patterns

"What Is My ADHD Like?"

SESSION SUMMARY

Overview

The theme of this session is developing mindful awareness of ADHD patterns and encouraging participants to ask themselves "What is my ADHD like?" What's new about this question is that participants are learning how to ask this question in an open and curious manner that encourages letting go of previous assumptions of what ADHD is and how it plays out in their daily lives. Emphasis is placed on nonjudgmental and compassionate self-observation in daily moments when ADHD behavior shows up. As part of this direct self-observation, difficulties in practicing meditation such as distractibility, restlessness, and boredom are discussed. These difficulties are presented as common for everyone, but also with recognition that they may be particularly difficult for those with ADHD. Such framing of ADHD as an extreme along a normal continuum of functioning discourages any feelings of separateness or defectiveness often voiced by individuals with ADHD. At the same time, while difficulties are explained and validated, participants are encouraged to work with the difficulties as much as they can and take responsibility for their actions. For example, in dealing with the difficulty of frequent distractions, it is emphasized that it is not about staying with, but about returning to the breath. In this way, the MT teaches participants to accept that (1) distraction will occur, (2) they can do something about it, and (3) they can persist in the effort of self-correction without harsh self-criticism. In this context, an acceptance–change dialectical approach is introduced as a universal framework to personal growth: participants can accept that difficulties can occur, while at the same time, participants can work to change the frequency and impact of these behaviors in the future. This is similar to the attitude used in cognitive-behavioral therapy for ADHD and ADHD coaching where gentle yet firm support is used to help with discouragement, lack of persistence, or inconsistent effort often reported in ADHD. At this session, mindfulness of movement and how ADHD is experienced in the body is also introduced—a concept that will be further addressed in the following sessions.

Session Outline

1) Brief opening meditation exercise: Counting Meditation (*Exercise 2.1*)
2) Review
    - Content of previous session
    - At-home practice experiences
3) Session theme: Common difficulties in practicing mindful awareness
    - Introduce the acceptance–change dialectic
4) Brief meditation exercise: Mindfulness of Breath (5 minutes) (*Exercise 2.2*)
5) Break
6) Mindfulness of movement
    - Mindful Standing and Balancing (*Exercise 2.3*)
    - Mindfulness of Walking (10 minutes) (*Exercise 2.4*)
7) Closing
    - Discussion of home practice
    - Brief Appreciation Meditation (*Exercise 2.5*)

Home Practice

1) Formal mindfulness practice: Mindfulness of Breath (5 minutes per day). Use optional Handout 2.1 to record noted difficulties and come up with potential solutions.
2) Informal mindfulness practice:
    - Noticing one's own ADHD symptoms with curiosity

BRIEF OPENING MEDITATION EXERCISE: COUNTING MEDITATION

This session sets a repeating pattern of having a brief meditation at the start of each session. The brief meditation exercise is typically tied to a practice learned in the previous session and serves as a reminder of the last week's concepts. This opening practice also helps participants to quiet down, relax into the meeting, and become more present.

COUNTING MEDITATION (5 MINUTES) (EXERCISE 2.1)

This opening exercise is similar to the Mindfulness of Breath exercise from the previous session, but this time participants are asked to count their breaths. Here's a script of how the MT might lead the group through this exercise:

> [*Ring bell.*]
>
> In this practice, we start by finding a comfortable sitting position. Keeping your back straight yet relaxed, as if you are sitting in a posture of dignity. Placing your hands on your lap or beside you.
>
> You may close your eyes or keep them half closed and resting in one spot, whichever way feels natural to you. As with last week's practice, find your breath in one spot, either the nostrils, chest, or belly. Noticing the movement of your belly, your chest, or the sensation of air moving in and out of your nostrils. If you're unsure of which spot you should choose, simply pick one and try it out this time. Any of these options are fine.
>
> In this practice, we are invited to count our breaths. A breath has two parts: one that involves breathing in the air around you and the other that involves breathing out. Take an in-breath, briefly hold it, then breathe out. Good, that's one breath. If you find yourself getting caught up on how you're breathing, just remember that there's no right or wrong way to do it. However your breath is right now is exactly where it should be.
>
> To count your breath, when you breathe in and out, silently, in your mind, say "one" to yourself. For the next breath, say "two" to yourself, then "three," then "four," and so on. If you get distracted and forget your number, simply start at the beginning again. Be curious how high you can count before I start to talk.
>
> [*Pause for 1 minute.*]
>
> Good, now notice "How far did I get?," "Did my mind get distracted?," "How far did I get until I got distracted?" Are you surprised by what you observed?
>
> Now I'm going to ring the bell to end the meditation. Listen to the whole sound of the bell. When you cannot hear it anymore, open your eyes.
>
> [*Ring bell.*]

The MT invites the participants to share their experience with the above practice and uses their comments to guide the discussion. This breath-counting exercise is often perceived as being easier to focus on than the practice of "just paying attention to the breath" because active counting can anchor the mind on the experience of breathing and counteract distractibility. Participants often report that counting gives their mind "something to do" that helps them stay focused on the exercise and resist distraction. For those who make this observation after the exercise, the MT can encourage curiosity about how this practice contrasts with the Mindfulness of Breath practice they were assigned in the previous session. The MT can also extrapolate on other ways to help anchor attention, such as imagery of the breath (i.e., imagining a wave or color coming in and out of the body with each breath) or using words like *in* for the in-breath and *out* for the out-breath. Another strategy, following instructions of a well-known mindfulness teacher, Thich Nhat Hanh, is to narrate the whole experience of breathing: "Breathing in, I know I am breathing in. Breathing out, I know I am breathing out." Participants are encouraged to investigate different ways to conduct the Mindfulness of Breathing practice and find a way(s) that is helpful to them.

REVIEW

Content of Previous Session

Briefly remind participants of the content discussed in the previous session. For example, "After introductions, we discussed what ADHD is, based on what we know from the research literature. We also discussed how ADHD shows up in daily life—a topic we'll build on today. We also provided an introduction to mindfulness, which included a discussion of what the research literature says about mindfulness treatments for adults with ADHD, as well as attention and the five senses and an introduction to mindfulness exercises (i.e., mindful eating and Mindfulness of Breath)." Finally, remind participants of the at-home practice.

At the start of the review, encourage participants to pull out any of the handout sheets from the previous session to help them with recalling details of last week and any questions they may have had since then. The previous session's handouts include: group rules, defining mindfulness, the concept of being on automatic pilot, and a home practice sheet to self-monitor how often they engaged in the at-home practices.

At this point, it is also important to help participants practice embodying the non-judgmental, curious attitude of mindfulness when recalling the previous week. For example, asking "Thinking about your experiences, are you noticing any judgmental or critical thoughts?" can also remind participants that sometimes the certainty people experience in negative judgments (e.g., "I'm no good at meditation") makes it more difficult to be open and curious. Discuss how openness to questioning previous assumptions and simply watching thoughts as "events" that may or may not be correct can help with building meta-awareness.

At-Home Practice Experiences

Ask participants to share their experience of doing the formal and informal mindfulness practices at home since the previous session. Remind them that it might be helpful to look at the handout sheet provided at the previous session or any other method they used to track their practice. The discussion is done in a way to allow for sharing, even if the participants were not able to do much weekly practice. The following questions are asked to facilitate the review, starting with the informal practice (since informal practice may have been easier for participants to do during the week):

Question Examples

- "How many of you practiced taking a mindful breath before picking up the phone?"
- "How many of you practiced mindfulness of a routine activity?"
- "How many times did you practice the formal Mindfulness of Breath exercise?"

For those who did the formal practice:

- "How many days per week?"

For all of these prompts, ask for more details:

- "What was your experience?"

Acknowledge the difficulties that participants encountered and validate these experiences. This might include making comments like, "It's common for these kinds of difficulties to pop up, especially as you're getting started." Balance out these types of comments with firm encouragement to continue practicing at home. Essentially, the MT is communicating to participants to *take the suggested practice seriously and challenge themselves, but also to (1) be kind to themselves if they did not practice, (2) be curious what got in the way of practice, and (3) practice mindfulness in their lives in whatever way is possible for them.*

During this discussion—ideally expanding on the sharing offered by the members of the group—clarify common misconceptions about mindfulness practices. Table S2.1 lists some common misconceptions and how to respond.

We encourage the MT to think about the participant's first week as the baseline that they're going to be working from and use the behavioral principle of shaping to guide participants. That is, shaping refers to reinforcing behaviors that are approaching and becoming successively closer to the behavioral goal. For example, if a participant practiced the Mindfulness of Breath exercise for 1 day in the past week, then verbally reinforce

TABLE S2.1. Common Misconceptions in Practicing Mindful Awareness

Misconception	MT's response
"I should be able to stay focused during the exercise, but I just can't."	"Getting distracted is common, especially as you're just learning this skill. It's not about whether you get distracted, but instead how you respond to yourself when you get distracted during the exercise (e.g., letting go of self-critical thinking and 'gently returning attention to the breath'). You could say, 'The practice is more about returning to the breath then staying with the breath,' and 'Every time you return to the breath, you are training your attention and awareness . . . like training the attention muscle.' "
"I couldn't empty my mind."	"Mindfulness is about being aware of what your experience is versus creating a specific experience. It involves focusing attention on a selected experience or object in the moment (e.g., breath) and then observing the process. Emptying or quieting of the mind may or may not happen, in fact often we first become more aware of how busy the mind really is during mindfulness practice."
"I didn't feel better afterward, so I must have been doing it wrong."	"It helps to simply be curious about the practice and what happens moment to moment versus a specific outcome. It's important that you set an intention to practice and then notice the process. Sometimes difficult feelings bubble up or you may notice increased restlessness. The purpose of the practice is to train awareness of what is—even unpleasant experiences. Ultimately, we learn how to be with, work with, or let these negative experience pass with equanimity."

them the next week if they practice for 2 days—in the long term, we want the practice to be more frequent, but in the short term an increase is getting closer to the long-term goal. For this session, assuming participants did not start already practicing mindfulness, any practice is more than before and therefore worth praising in the session.

An additional facet of homework completion is quality versus quantity. When the MT asks about practice frequency and duration, they're focusing on quantity. However, the quality of the practice should not be ignored because it can be just as important. For example, from the Practice Quality-Mindfulness Questionnaire (Del Re, Fluckiger, Goldberg, & Hoyt, 2013) ask questions such as:

Question Examples

- "During practice, did you attempt to return to each experience, no matter how unpleasant, with a sense that 'It's okay to experience this?' "
- "During practice, were you actively avoiding or 'pushing away' certain experiences?"
- "During practice, were you actively trying to fix or change certain experiences in order to get to a 'better place?' "

We recommend inclusion of questions along these lines to draw out the quality of participant experiences and point out this aspect of mindfulness practice for them.

ADAPTATION TO INDIVIDUAL THERAPY

Much of what is discussed during review can largely follow what's outlined here. However, with individual therapy there's more time to explore individual experiences. The MT may, for example, help the individual more closely monitor their at-home practice in the form of visual feedback (e.g., graphs) to establish a baseline for practice that can be referenced in future sessions.

SESSION THEME: COMMON DIFFICULTIES IN PRACTICING MINDFUL AWARENESS

The main theme of this session is **common difficulties that arise in practicing mindful awareness**, particularly during formal mindfulness meditation exercises. Drawing on the discussion of the previous week's practice, prompt the participants to take a couple of minutes and use Handout 2.1 to list such difficulties. After the short reflection, ask participants to share what difficulties they experienced and write these on the board. The discussion that follows should list not only common difficulties that arise during meditation, but how they overlap with ADHD. For example, distractibility, restlessness, and boredom are common in ADHD. Table S2.2 lists some typical examples of difficulties that commonly arise and potential solutions.

As you identify these solutions to common meditation difficulties, also ask participants to reflect on the common ADHD struggles discussed in the previous session. In many cases, given the nature of ADHD, the difficulties experienced in practice are to be expected and frequent. To encourage perseverance, reframe difficulties as

TABLE S2.2. Common Difficulties and Solutions for Practicing Mindful Awareness

Difficulties	Solution
Distraction during the exercise	Getting distracted is common, especially when one begins practicing mindfulness. Further, this is a core symptom of ADHD, so it just might take more time and practice. Also, think about gradually getting better over time. Remind participants to practice being kind to themselves and that mindfulness is not about perfection, but intention to focus and renewing that intention each time they catch themselves getting distracted.
Falling asleep during the exercise	Tell participants to choose a time of day to practice in which they're more awake (e.g., just after their morning coffee). Another solution is to ask what their body posture was: Were they sitting up in a dignified, attentive pose, or laying down in bed? The latter is going to be more conducive to falling asleep. Another way to enhance wakefulness might be to keep their eyes open during an exercise or to do a mindfulness exercise that allows for movement.
Forget to practice	Prompt participants to use visual reminders (e.g., a Post-it Note) or auditory reminders (e.g., an alarm on a phone). Remind them to find a "mindfulness buddy"—just like an "exercise buddy," they remind you and encourage you to practice.
Feel unmotivated or bored	Participants should choose a time of the day when they're more likely to feel motivated. Another solution is to use the Premack principle, which refers to using a higher-probability behavior to serve as a reinforcer for a lower-probability behavior (e.g., if you enjoy tea, have a cup of tea *after* you practice a formal mindfulness meditation). Another recommendation is arrange one's environment to make it easier to practice (i.e., modifying an antecedent to change the probability of a behavior to occur). For example, it can be helpful to designate an area in one's home as a meditation spot. Relatedly, have visual reminders for practice (meditation pillow, a picture that is a personal reminder of intention for practice, a candle), which may serve as discriminative stimuli consistent with the phenomenon of stimulus control. While typical mindfulness practice does not call for music, lighting of candles, or another ritual, it may be helpful and motivating to incorporate such elements. As the MT, guide participants to bring curiosity to how they are experiencing the different elements of their practice and its impact on motivation. Finally, invite participants to explore what they notice about the feeling of boredom itself. For example, what do they notice in their body or their thoughts when they feel bored?
Could not sit still/restlessness	Suggest that participants try a walking meditation (practiced in this session) or practice sitting meditation after having done some physical exertion, exercise, or another body-relaxing activity (e.g., being in the sauna). Alternatively, encourage participants to see if they can "hold" the restlessness from a wider perspective (tolerating it for some time as "just a sensation to notice"), breathe more deeply, and/or encourage body to relax or let go of restlessness before shifting to an exercise that allows for movement.

(continued)

TABLE S2.2. *(continued)*

Difficulties	Solution
Second-guessing or doubtful thoughts about one's ability to practice mindfulness	Remind participants that thoughts are thoughts—no more, no less. Encourage them to watch the doubting thoughts the same way they would watch other thoughts. Remind participants to be patient and kind with themselves and "Let your experience be your guide as you learn this new skill."
Second-guessing or doubtful thoughts about the utility of meditation that create an aversion to practice	Remind participants about the original intention to practice mindfulness and the long-term improvements it can provide. Suggest that they bring curiosity to their current experience and adopt "a witness perspective," noting that their thoughts, including doubting thoughts, come and go while they continue to practice.
Craving or wanting to experience mindfulness meditation in a certain way	Sometimes we expect to experience a mindfulness meditation in a certain way (e.g., to feel a greater sense of peace or stillness), but we don't reach that desired outcome in a particular session. In those cases, remind participants to "let go" of judgments they have about how the exercise should be—instead remind them that they are setting an intention to practice. Anything beyond that may be out of their control. Can they accept that the experience they have for that exercise is going to be the experience they have—no more, no less? Encourage participants to recognize that the craving often creates more suffering than the experience itself.

"opportunities to practice awareness." Ask participants to actively observe their own experiences nonjudgmentally, discuss how the ADHD symptoms are on a continuum, and engage with these difficulties with a curiosity about their own ADHD (i.e., "What is my ADHD like?"). One guiding framework during this conversation is that MTs can support participants by modeling a curious and empathic response when adult ADHD behaviors create difficulty. This type of MT support can provide guidance on how to approach one's own experience in a way that balances acceptance and change, which is elaborated upon in the next section.

Introduce the Acceptance–Change Dialectic

The discussion of difficulties is a good springboard to discuss the acceptance–change dialectic (as originally described in DBT). Many participants will likely come to treatment with behavioral, emotional, and cognitive concerns related to their ADHD, with a change-oriented outlook. For example, they may struggle with focusing on a task and often become distracted by extraneous stimuli. With a change-oriented outlook, they may expect therapy to teach skills that can reduce these occurrences. However, similar to approaches like DBT (Linehan, 1993) and ACT (Hayes et al., 2012), the MAPs for ADHD Program tries to counterbalance this change-oriented approach with one of acceptance. For example, the MT may comment in the following way: "The mindfulness techniques can be used to help manage ADHD behaviors, such as restlessness or noticing when your attention has strayed. However, just as this can be helpful, it is important to find a balance between change and acceptance. For instance, can you imagine how trying to change feeling restless might actually cause more restlessness for you?" As you elicit feedback from participants, look for discussion points that involve where acceptance of restlessness (or being bored, frustrated, distracted, overwhelmed, etc.) might be more skillful than attempting to change this state. Point out how accepting something first, paves a way for a helpful change later. For example, participants may at times tell themselves they shouldn't feel what they feel in the moment—leading to emotional avoidance or self-critical thoughts. Point out that pushing away a feeling can make it stay around longer, while acceptance of the feeling, allowing yourself to have the feeling, can help diffuse or regulate the feeling. Another example is difficulty focusing after getting little sleep or after an emotionally intense experience and learning to accept the current limitation rather than attempting to change it. With these or other examples, you are attempting to get participants to entertain the idea that both change and acceptance perspectives are needed. This discussion should include the following aspects about the acceptance–change dialectic:

First, acceptance is an important initial step of behavior change, even though it's the opposite of change. This is not passively accepting things and "having to like them," but it is a stance of more radical allowing and acknowledging things as they are in the moment, including those things you may not want. A mindfulness-based approach teaches that by nonjudgmentally accepting (or allowing) "what is" in the moment, new choices for skillful responding likely become available.

Second, point out how the initial acceptance leads to discernment about what is the next skillful step. Sometimes what's needed is acceptance that something cannot be changed; other times what's needed is proactive action to change something. This last point also involves an underlying assumption of the MAPs for ADHD Program—when participants are able to observe their own behavior and experiences, they can use mindfulness training as a platform to choose how they respond. Thus, mindfulness training does not tell them how to respond, rather it teaches the process of responding. The MT assumes that participants will make the more skillful decisions when they apply mindfulness techniques.

Third, remind participants to adopt a nonjudgmental perspective and help them to that end by acknowledging the universality of human struggles. Discuss that if ADHD symptoms are on a continuum, as was discussed in Session 1, than others—even those without ADHD—experience similar difficulties from time to time. Encourage participants to avoid comparing themselves to others, criticizing themselves for having a particular experience, or pushing negative thoughts or feelings away. Acknowledge that it can feel aversive to accept things you don't want. Remind participants that their old behavioral repertoire may be to avoid things that are aversive. With therapy, we ask them to try something new, which may even be the opposite of what they typically do. In this case, as opposed to avoidance, we are asking them to approach some aversive states when they practice acceptance. This may result in "short-term pain for long-term gain."

ADAPTATION TO INDIVIDUAL THERAPY

The MT has more time to focus on developing more individualized solutions when using Table S2.2. Many of these solutions can build off principles of behavior change, such as modifying antecedents and consequences to impact behavior. In this case, the behavior is formal mindfulness meditation. As listed in Table S2.2, choosing a time of the day in which participants are more awake is an example of modifying an antecedent to change the likelihood of a behavior occurring. Use of the Premack principle described there is an example of modifying consequences to change the likelihood of that behavior occurring again.

BRIEF MEDITATION EXERCISE: MINDFULNESS OF BREATH

MINDFULNESS OF BREATH (5 MINUTES) (EXERCISE 2.2)

This exercise is the same as Exercise 1.3 in Session 1 (see page 56); however, the participants are asked to actively notice any difficulties that arise during the meditation and notice how they respond to them. Building off of the difficulties that were acknowledged earlier in this session, remind them: *"It's not just about staying with your breath, but also returning to your breath when your mind gets off track."*

BREAK

This is approximately the midpoint in the session, where a 5- to 10-minute break is taken.

MINDFULNESS OF MOVEMENT

Early on in the MAPs for ADHD Program, we encourage teaching participants that not all mindfulness practices involve sitting still. Mindfulness can be brought to any state, including movement or daily activity. This "mindfulness practices require me to sit still all the time" misunderstanding is important to dispel, especially for those participants who are high in hyperactive-impulsive symptoms. We recommend leading with a brief discussion of ADHD symptoms and diverse presentations of the disorder. For example, fidgeting and difficulty staying seated are the first two hyperactive-impulsive symptoms listed in the DSM-5. The MT should point out that in teaching mindfulness, on the one hand, we want participants to challenge themselves and practice observing and being with (versus acting on) such difficult feelings. On the other hand, we want to balance that with the degree of difficulty they are experiencing while sitting. MT should discuss how mindful movement is an alternative to sitting still and empower each participant with the choice to get up during a sitting practice and do mindful walking instead when sitting is very difficult. In this way, the participants are also encouraged to practice kindness, self-care, and wise choices during practice.

Mindful movement is introduced via two practices: (1) Mindful Standing and Balancing and (2) Mindfulness of Walking exercises.[1]

[1] For those who are unable to participate in these movement exercises, such as participants with mobility issues, MTs are encouraged to adapt them to meet the needs of the group. For example, in Exercise 2.3, participants can perform this exercise while sitting and attempt to notice any movement while they attempt to sit still as opposed to stand still. See Chapter 3 for other suggestions.

MINDFUL STANDING AND BALANCING (EXERCISE 2.3)

Please stand up, push your chairs in, and stand behind your chairs.

This is going to be a gentle movement and stretching exercise. In this exercise, you'll be invited to become more aware of your bodily movement and sensations, which we'll continue to build on in future sessions.

Close your eyes or keep them resting in one spot.

Bring attention to your body. Notice your body standing up. Be curious and ask yourself "How am I standing?" and "What is my posture?" Without trying to change how you are standing, ask yourself, "Does my body feel different standing rather than when I was just sitting?" and, if so, "What do I notice?" If you don't notice any difference, that's perfectly fine—we're simply checking in about what you notice when you stand, and sometime that can be nothing at all.

Stand completely still. Try not to move your body at all. Is it possible to not move at all? Can you stand there without even moving one inch?

[*Pause for about 30 seconds of silence.*]

Were you able to stand perfectly still? Probably not. Our bodies are always in motion, even when we attempt to be still. However, we may not notice this because we haven't spent much time paying attention to this way we experience our bodies.

Now, start to *very slowly* shift your weight onto your right foot. You may want to hold on to your chair. Notice the sensation in your foot as your weight moves onto the right foot. When I say "sensation," I mean anything you can feel in your body. Now, shift your weight *very slowly* onto your left foot. Do you notice any teeny tiny sensations in your foot as your weight shifts from one side to the next?

Now shift back and forth at your own pace in a way that does not make you lose your balance or move your chair. I'm going to give you about 20 seconds to shift back and forth so that you can observe if you notice anything as you shift your weight.

Okay, now return to standing on both feet. Imagine your feet as firmly planted in the ground, almost like your legs are strong tree trunks firmly rooted in the ground beneath you. Imagine the strength of those roots working their way up your body. Does your posture feel more upright? Do you have a sense of height that you didn't have before? Can you imagine yourself being firmly rooted? Think about how you stood at the start of this exercise and how that has or hasn't changed. Take a moment to find your stance. See if you can find a sense of stillness, even though your body will continue to have small movements.

Bring your awareness back to your feet, take a deep breath, then open your eyes.

MINDFULNESS OF WALKING (10 MINUTES) (EXERCISE 2.4)

Participants will be standing at their chairs after the last exercise. Invite them to remain standing. Unlike exercises up until this point when the MT provides a rationale for the practice prior to it, in this exercise the MT will provide experiential learning prior to discussing its significance for ADHD. This is in part practical—participants are already standing. This is also purposeful—the MT wants to start modeling that the primary way to learn about mindfulness is experiential—learning through practice as opposed to learning through discussion. In the MAPs for ADHD Program, we recommend guiding the exercise at different rates of walking: slow, average, and fast (in contrast to classical mindful walking that is done in a slow deliberate way only).

Here's how the MT might narrate this exercise:

Let's form a circle and give the person next to you some room. Turn to your left so you are facing the back of the person next to you.

Go ahead and start walking.

[*Allow the group to make about one rotation, this serves as a reference point for "mindless walking" similar to how they might typically walk. Provide little guidance about speed, talking, or anything else.*]

Now stop and close your eyes. Let your body become more still and quiet. Feel your body standing—find your posture. Without trying to change anything, notice your weight and if there is any tension or pain, or maybe good feelings.

Good, now open your eyes. We are going to try a walking meditation in a circle. Whereas we just walked as we typically do, which we might call "typical" or perhaps "mindless walking," now we're going to focus on the sensations of moving your feet as a way of mindful walking. This might be a little more challenging because we all are walking together, so we have to pay attention to our neighbor so we don't step on their foot or have any collisions. Having someone close by during this exercise might also be an opportunity to practice mindfulness. That is, you may feel impatient, maybe because you want to walk faster or differently than the person in front of you. But we have to practice patience and stay with your own experience, so if you notice impatience or frustration emerging, remind yourself that it serves as a reminder to practice staying with the experience of walking.

Another thing is what to do with your eyes. Obviously, we don't want to walk around with our eyes closed. Narrow your gaze in front of you so that you can minimize seeing things that may distract you, while being able to see well enough to walk without running into others. Avoid looking around, as it can be distracting; however, keep yourself aware of where you are going. We are going to do this walk silently, without talking or making noises. We're going to begin purposefully walking slowly. Ready? Let's begin.

As you start to walk, slowly lift one of your legs and begin to walk. In your mind, you can label the movement as "lifting and placing" "lifting and placing," or simply observe your movement without labeling.

As you walk slowly, do you notice any teeny tiny sensations in your feet and legs? What about the sensations of your feet touching the ground? The placement of the ball of the foot and the shift in weight and balance as you walk? Be curious and open about your experience. Stay connected to the sensations of walking.

You may want to experiment and see what it's like to synchronize your breathing with your footsteps. For example, as you step with one foot, inhale; as you step with the other foot, exhale. Do whatever most closely matches between the pace of your breathing and your walking.

When your mind wanders, congratulate yourself for catching it wandering. Then, gently give yourself permission to bring your attention back to the sensations in the soles of your feet. Do this as often as your mind wanders—there's no limit and there's no such thing as catching yourself too much.

[*Allow participants to walk slowly in silence for 30–60 seconds.*]

Where is your attention right now? If you need to, bring it back to lifting and placing your feet.

Notice the movement of your entire leg or arms instead of the sensations of your feet. As you slow down, gradually narrow your focus back to your feet.

Stop walking. Close your eyes. Use this as an opportunity to stop and feel your whole body. How many parts of your body you can notice? Bring your sensation to how you feel emotionally on the inside. Is there is a sense of impatience? Frustration? Wanting to rush? A sense of relaxation? Simply notice whatever your experience is with openness, kindness, and curiosity. Let go of any judgments you have about these experiences. They are already here and you can let them be.

[*Repeat these instructions for practicing going at a medium pace, then a fast pace.*]

As we end, see if you can bring a sense of gratefulness for your body for its ability to carry and support you throughout each day, as well as your willingness to stop and check in with it.

[*Pause and then ring bell.*]

Check in with participants on how the practice went for them. You may want to ask questions to elicit discussion about the exercise, such as:

Question Examples

- "What was it like to walk slowly all together at the same time without talking?"
- "What was difficult about walking that way?"
- "Did you want to walk differently than the person in front of you?"
- "Did you notice your [insert body part, such as feet, legs, arms] while you were walking?"
- "What kinds of things did you notice that we haven't discussed yet?"

This discussion will often address how ADHD is experienced in the body, setting a foundation for later sessions. Participants may be unclear how movement applies to ADHD in particular. In fact, we would expect this to be the case, since ADHD and bodily movements/sensations are not typically discussed together. Ask participants if they have any thoughts on this based on the exercise they just completed—how can ADHD and movement be related? The MT will want to introduce how clumsiness from core symptoms, such as making careless mistakes or failing to pay close attention to detail, may be applicable. Or, the MT may ask participants about times they are late and the speed at which they move their bodies. Do they ever move so quickly because they're pressed for time that they put something down and later can't remember where they put it? Were they not attending to the bodily movements they engaged in while setting things down?

The mindfulness of movement exercises also allow for participants to resist fighting against the urge to move. These types of exercises allow participants to accept their restlessness and respond to it in a different way. For participants who gravitate toward these exercises, ask them to be curious about other ways to practice mindfulness during physical movement.

One adaptation to explore is having participants draw out the rhythm of their breath during the Mindfulness of Breath exercise. See Figure S2.1 for an example. In this example, each in-breath is drawn as the line ascending and the out-breath as the line descending. You can see in this example how breathing started out faster, but then slowed down. Explore how this adaptation provides an outlet for not wanting to move

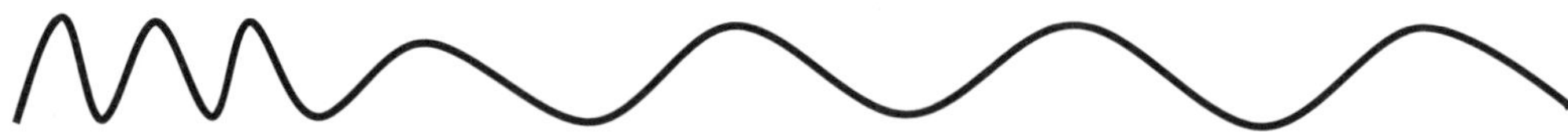

FIGURE S2.1. Example of drawing the rhythm of the breath during a mindfulness of breath exercise. The visual can help participants have realistic expectations during the practice (e.g., his or her breath may not slow down right away and he or she may not feel relaxed right away). Also, such incorporation of drawing during a sitting may be more engaging to some participants who otherwise struggle with hyperactive-impulsive symptoms. Those with predominantly inattentive symptoms may find that drawing helps focus, anchoring their attention to the practice.

or a tendency to lose focus. For those participants who view their hyperactive-impulsive symptoms as an impediment toward mindfulness practice, this adaptation can teach that one can "move with, instead of struggle against symptoms" and observe the experience mindfully. For those participants who struggle with inattention, drawing can anchor their attention to the practice. You can make a connection between this exercise and doodling, which some members may recognize as their own strategy for dealing with restlessness, inattention, or boredom.

ADAPTATION TO INDIVIDUAL THERAPY

The MT may spend more time collaborating with their patient on adapting the mindfulness exercises taught thus far. Examples include: (1) placing hand on the stomach to feel the breath during a mediation practice; (2) variations on the counting meditation, such as simply counting one (in-breath)—two (out-breath), one (in-breath)—two (out-breath) and so on; and (3) noticing the movement of arms and the breathing while walking. In this way, the MT and the patient can design an at-home practice that is doable for the individual patient.

CLOSING

Discussion of Home Practice

The MT should make sure to take sufficient time to review the plan for exercises to complete at home. This is more than simply summarizing what their tasks are, but instead it is time to address questions, clarify any points of confusion, and "fill in the blanks" for any participants who may have experienced mind wandering during parts of the session or those who feel unsure about what is being asked of them in the week ahead. The following are the basic points to convey (also summarized in Handout 2.2).

Continue the 5-minute Mindfulness of Breath exercise each day as the formal practice. Ensure that participants have picked a time and place each day that is conducive to successfully meeting this goal. Track difficulties that emerge while engaging in the exercise each day and write them in the last column (i.e., Comments). Participants can also use Handout 2.1 to record noted difficulties and come up with potential solutions.

For informal practice this week, observe your own ADHD symptoms with curiosity in daily life. Up to this point, the MT has provided participants with enough ADHD education so that they know what to look for and also the language to describe it in a nonjudgmental way. Some participants may wish to use something other than the handout provided in the session. For example, participants may wish to create journal entries and provide more contexts about their ADHD. The medium for documenting this practice in observing one's own ADHD is less important than them gaining the knowledge about how ADHD plays out for them on a day-to-day basis. As an option, Handout 2.3 may be used as well.

BRIEF APPRECIATION MEDITATION (EXERCISE 2.5)

At the close of this session, introduce a short meditation lasting about 2 minutes that includes a moment to stop and reflect on the session just completed and appreciation for participants, including themselves. A similar brief closing practice is used at the end of each subsequent session. Invite participants to offer appreciation or loving-kindness to themselves for making the time to practice mindfulness and self-care, and offer appreciation to others for their presence in the class. The short closing meditation allows participants to experience positive emotions and gratefulness. Here's how the exercise might be narrated:

> We close with a short appreciation practice. Sit in a relaxed yet upright posture and either close your eyes or keep them resting in one spot.
>
> [*Ring bell.*]
>
> Take a moment to appreciate everyone's presence today. People attending the group are here to care for themselves or to better their situations. The reasons may differ, but everyone is here to grow and improve their lives. Also, bring a sense of appreciation to yourself, for being here and taking the time for learning about yourself and mindfulness. See if you can connect with a sense of appreciation and gratitude in your body as you offer it to others and yourself.
>
> [*Ring bell.*]

Depending on factors like the amount of time left in the session, for a slightly longer version of this exercise that incorporates components of loving-kindness mindfulness meditation, you may want to incorporate the following into the exercise above:

> In your mind, say the following to others: "May you be happy, may you be safe, may you be healthy and live with ease." *[Repeat this line two or three more times.]*
>
> Avoid forcing a sense of appreciation. Instead, simply ask yourself if it's there already. If it's not there, just setting the intention to appreciate the presence of others is important.
>
> Now, take a moment and offer yourself loving-kindness for making the time to practice mindfulness and take care of yourself, which will then help you take care of others and situations once you walk out of this room.
>
> In your mind, say the following to yourself: "May I be happy, may I be safe, may I be healthy and live with ease." *[Repeat this line two or three more times.]*
>
> Take this feeling of appreciation with you, but before you mentally leave the room, take this moment to sit and allow yourself to experience the positive emotion and a sense of gratefulness.

Let it spread in your body and move outward with you as you move on to the next part of your day.

[*Ring bell.*]

The weekly Home Practice Sheet (Handout 2.2) is given at the end of session. If the MT decides to send weekly email summaries after the group is completed, please refer to the end of Session 1 for an example of the structure of those emails. Also, see Session 1 for adaptation for individual therapy.

SESSION 3

Mindful Awareness of Sound, Breath, and Body

SESSION SUMMARY

Overview

In this session, participants explore sound, breath, and body sensations as *the three anchors to the present moment.* Different practices are introduced to explore paying attention to these anchors and noticing shifts between them. While attentional movement from one stimulus to the next is often familiar to the ADHD individual, being aware of the changing of attention from an "impartial observer" stance or intentionally directing such shifts is often a new experience. Mindful awareness of sound is introduced using a short musical piece during which the participants are asked to observe their experience of listening, including shifts of attention to different instruments, evoked feelings, imagery, or thought associations. Additional sound awareness is practiced using the meditation bell. Mindful Standing and Stretching practice serves as a way to explore attention to diverse body sensations. This is followed by a silent meditation during which the participants are asked to pay attention to the shifts between the three anchors of ambient sound, breath, or body sensation. At the close of the session, the participants are asked to practice mindful awareness throughout the week by using cueing questions of "Where is my attention right now?" or "What am I doing right now?" and bringing themselves back to the intended task. Visual reminders, such as sticker dots or a frame with the word "breathe," are recommended as external reminders to connect with present moment awareness. Use of external reminders is adapted from a CBT approach for ADHD (Safren, Perlman, Sprich, & Otto, 2005) in this way to make it applicable in the context of mindfulness practices.

Session Outline

1) Brief opening meditation exercise: Mindfulness of Breath (*Exercise 3.1*)
2) Review
   - Content of previous session
   - At-home practice experiences
3) Session theme: Noticing shifts in attention and body awareness
4) Mindful Awareness of Music (*Exercise 3.2*)
5) Mindfulness of Sound (*Exercise 3.3*)
6) Mindful Standing and Stretching (*Exercise 3.4*)
7) Break
8) Mindfulness of Sound, Breath, and Body (*Exercise 3.5*)
9) S.T.O.P. Introduction and Practice (*Exercise 3.6*)
10) Closing
    - Discussion of home practice
    - Brief Appreciation Meditation (*Exercise 3.7*)

Home Practice

1) Formal mindfulness practice: Mindfulness of Sound, Breath, and Body (10 minutes per day)
2) Informal mindfulness practice:
   - Sound and walking or S.T.O.P. practice
   - Attention check-in: "Where is my attention right now?," "What am I doing right now?," and using visual reminders

BRIEF OPENING MEDITATION EXERCISE: MINDFULNESS OF BREATH

Similar to the previous session and for the remainder of treatment, start with a brief meditation exercise that attempts to tie in an aspect of the practice learned the previous week. This exercise typically lasts about 5 minutes. For this opening exercise, the main aim is to review the previous session's focus on the breath and difficulties that arise in sitting practice. This brief Mindfulness of Breath is guided by the MT. The opening practice also helps participants to quiet down, relax into the meeting, and become more present.

MINDFULNESS OF BREATH (EXERCISE 3.1)

[*Ring bell.*]

Find a relaxed and comfortable sitting position. Keep your back straight and relaxed as if you are sitting in a posture of dignity. Place your hands on your lap or by your side.

Close your eyes or keep them half closed and resting in one spot.

In this practice, we will be focusing and staying with your breath for the next few minutes.

Take a deep breath and allow yourself to simply rest in the present moment.

Let your usual preoccupations or need to do something else fall into the background.

Find a spot where it is easy for you to feel your breath—either your nostrils, chest, or belly.

Bring in your full attention and notice the natural flow of air coming in . . . and going out.

No need to change your breathing, simply noticing your breath as it is naturally.

Notice the transition points between the in-breath and the out-breath. Those points are points of stillness and pause. Notice how your body initiates each breath cycle . . . in a way, how the body breathes itself. See if you can rest and watch the breathing happening naturally, automatically, and perhaps even bring a sense of gratefulness to how the body takes care of the breathing for you.

We will practice this in silence for a few minutes. Remember, if your mind wanders off 100 times, gently bring it back to your breath 100 times.

[*Ring bell.*]

REVIEW

Content of Previous Session

Briefly remind participants of the content discussed in the previous session—for example, "Recall that last session we talked about developing a mindful awareness of your ADHD patterns and asking yourself 'What is my ADHD like?' in an open, curious, compassionate, and nonjudgmental manner." Additional points for this discussion include: (1) reframing ADHD as an extreme along a normal continuum of functioning; (2) responding to interfering ADHD without self-criticism and practicing reorienting toward the originally intended focus; and (3) introducing the Mindfulness of Movement exercises.

At-Home Practice Experiences

The MT asks each participant to report on their experience of doing at-home practice during the week, especially noting difficulties and ADHD-related behaviors. Participants are asked to review their tracking sheets and share their experience with the group. The difficulties may include getting to practice at all or an unwanted experience during the silent practice. The acceptance–change dialectic is recalled as a way to motivate participants to continue engaging with mindfulness without shaming or criticizing themselves if they have not yet practiced at home.

SESSION THEME: NOTICING SHIFTS IN ATTENTION AND BODY AWARENESS

The main theme of this session is exploring attentional shifts between three different objects of attention: sound, breath, and body sensations. These three objects are discussed as *the three anchors to the present moment* (see Figure S3.1).

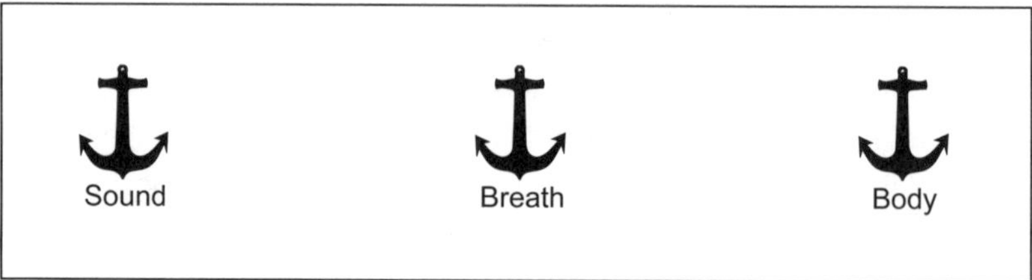

FIGURE S3.1. Three anchors to the present moment.

The anchors are places where attention can be directed when a person feels distracted, is lost in thinking or rumination, or is simply behaving in an automatic, not fully aware way. Participants will be familiar with their attention straying from one thing to the next and not being fully present in the moment, which are common experiences in ADHD. What's likely going to be new for participants is the message that they can use mindfulness techniques to be more aware of these shifts in attention and that they can be "in the driver's seat" of where their attention goes. As the MT elicits examples from participants about how their attention strays from the present moment during times their ADHD is more apparent to them, the MT describes how attention can be highjacked and how coming back to the three anchors can strengthen the attentional muscle. The three anchors are discussed as "always there and available to us to become more present." Different practices are introduced to explore paying attention to these anchors and playing with shifts between them. The MT discusses that distraction or "spacing out" is often familiar to those with ADHD, but being aware of the "grabbing" and intentionally directing such shifts is often a new experience.

MINDFUL AWARENESS OF MUSIC

To allow participants to experientially learn about their attention shifts, we recommend the following music exercise. Participants are asked to purposefully shift their focus from one thing to the next during the exercise. The exploration of sounds is introduced via a musical piece about 2–3 minutes in length. There are no specific directions on what type of music the MT should play, although we recommend it be instrumental with a number of different instruments that can be heard individually.

MINDFUL AWARENESS OF MUSIC (EXERCISE 3.2)

Our intention here is to train our focus and alertness. When we listen to music, we're listening for the moment-to-moment changes and shifts in the sound rather than being "swept up by the music."

I am going to play you a piece. [*Start music.*] See if you can listen to it with complete attention. As you're listening, notice what happens to your attention. When does it wander off? Where does it go? Don't get too analytical. Practice noticing and coming back to the sounds as fully as you possibly can.

Notice if you can direct your attention to one instrument for a minute (e.g., the drums, piano, guitar, horns), then shift your awareness to a different instrument.

Observe any changes in tempo or intensity.

Does the music evoke any feelings, thoughts, or imagery for you?

Do you notice any body responses to the music?

The MT invites the participants to *share their experiences with the above practice* and uses their comments to guide the discussion. During this discussion, the MT inquires if participants were able to shift their focus from one instrument to another. If so, how was such purposeful focus different from automatic pilot mode? During the conversation, the MT attempts to guide participants to consider how this type of experience might be relevant in the context of their ADHD symptoms.

MINDFULNESS OF SOUND

The exploration of sound from the exercise above is continued with awareness of a simple or pure sound using a meditation bell. The MT explains how the previous exercise gave the participants something specific to listen to (i.e., the music). In this exercise, after listening to the sound of a bell, participants will practice listening to whatever sounds are in their environment without directing their attention to one specific source.

MINDFULNESS OF SOUND (EXERCISE 3.3)

Keep your eyes open. I am going to ring a bell. When I ring the bell, listen to the sound until you hear it has stopped ringing. Raise your hand when you can no longer hear the bell.

[*Ring bell and allow period of silence to follow. Let participants notice how long it took each other to notice the absence of the bell.*]

Now we are going to try the same exercise with our eyes closed, and this time, listen as attentively as you can and put up your hand when you no longer hear the sound of the bell. Close your eyes—let your body be still and quiet. Don't open up your eyes at all.

[*Ring bell and allow silence until last participant has put up his or her hand.*]

Good. Were you more or less attentive when your eyes were closed? Could you hear the bell, even when it was very quiet and barely audible?

We're going to continue listening, but not to the bell. Keep your eyes closed and listen to the sounds in the room or outside the room. Just listen, don't label what the sounds are yet. The sounds could be in your body or outside your body. Don't do anything special but pay attention to sound. You don't have to seek out any particular sounds—simply let them come to you. [*Pause 15 seconds.*] See if you can listen to the sound without making up a story about the sound. You may hear a cough and think, "Oh, I wonder who coughed, and I wonder if they are sick, and maybe I'll get sick, and so on." You can make up a lot of stories about sound, but see if you can listen to sounds without making up any story. Just listening. [*Pause 30 seconds.*]

Now I will ring the bell to end our meditation time. Wait to open your eyes until the sound of the bell is completely gone and whenever I ring the bell in the future, see if you can listen to the whole sound of the bell like we did today. [*Ring bell.*]

After the exercise, the MT leads a discussion of the participants' experiences during the sound meditation. MT prompts could include:

- "Raise your hand if the bell sounded for a very long time."
- "Were you surprised that the bell's ring wasn't for a shorter duration?"
- "What sounds did you hear?"
- "What does ____________ [the sound observed] sound like?"
- "Did you seek the sounds out or did they just come to you?"
- "Did you start to make up stories about these sounds? How did you respond to yourself when you caught yourself caught up in a narrative—not the sound itself?"

The MT should remind participants that if they caught themselves getting distracted in any way during the exercise, to let go of any judgmental self-talk.

MINDFUL STANDING AND STRETCHING

Next, the MT introduces the anchor of body sensations. Breath is one such sensation the participants have already been focusing on, but in this practice, the attention is drawn to other body sensations that occur with movement. Remind participants that being mindful of body sensations is one of the three anchors that we are focusing on for this session. In our work, we typically practice Mindful Standing and Stretching for about 5 minutes, followed by a 2–3 minute discussion in which responses from participants are elicited.

MINDFUL STANDING AND STRETCHING (EXERCISE 3.4)

In this exercise we will explore movement and body sensations.

Please stand and invite yourself to become relaxed yet curious about your body in this position. Bring attention to your posture and notice how your body feels standing.

You may notice the point of contact with the ground, sensations of air on your face or hands, or perhaps some discomfort or pain in an area of your body.

If it helps you to connect with each sensation, you might quietly say in your mind, "tingling . . . pressure . . . pulsing . . . tensing . . . softening" or whatever label describes your experience in the moment.

Staying present, notice if and how the sensations change from moment to moment.

Now as you stand see if you can become perfectly still.

You may notice natural subtle movements even if your intention is to be still.

Now, move from side to side by shifting your weight from one leg to the other. Try that a few times and bring awareness to the sensations and the ways you keep yourself in balance.

Now, coming back to center, explore a subtle movement forward and backward with your body. Practice keeping yourself in balance and observing the body sensations during such movements.

Come back to the center again and this time, raise both arms slowly above your head, paying attention to the movement and the sensation of stretching. Lower your arms slowly and again notice the sense of movement, air, tingling, or feeling of blood flow in your arms. Repeat the up and down movement with awareness.

Finally, shake your hands for about 15 seconds and then stop. Observe the sensation in your hands.

ADAPTATION TO INDIVIDUAL THERAPY

The Mindful Standing and Stretching meditation can be practiced seated, without a need to change a typical way the patient interacts with the therapist. The instructions would be adapted to noticing sensations while sitting (e.g., if patient is sitting in a relaxed way, asking the patient to sit upright with back supported and noticing sensations in the body after such a positional shift). The therapist can also invite individual patients to interlace and stretch their fingers, raise and stretch their arms them above their head or shake their hands. As with the group exercise, the patient is asked to attend to the moment-by-moment changes in body sensations.

BREAK

This is approximately the midpoint in the session, where a 5- to 10-minute break is taken.

MINDFULNESS OF SOUND, BREATH, AND BODY

In this exercise, the MT asks the participants to sequentially focus on ambient sounds, then the breath, and then the body as a whole. This is a practice of setting intention to keeping attention/awareness on a chosen object (sound), then releasing the object and shifting attention to a new object (breath), and then again making another transition to a new object (other body sensation). As mentioned above, attentional movement from one stimulus to the next often happens automatically for the ADHD individual, and this exercise asks participants to be more intentional and directive (i.e., "in the driver seat") of the attention switches. After the experience of purposefully directing their attention to different domains of experience, the participants are asked to notice "what is predominant" from moment to moment (whether it is a breath, their body, a sound, or a thought). The breath or another anchor (sound or body) are emphasized as a place to return to whenever one becomes distracted or caught in thinking. This last part of the exercise, noticing where the attention goes spontaneously, further develops the meta-awareness experience of tracking attention.

For a visual depiction that may help the MT describe this exercise, we recommend describing this meditation analogous to the shape of our hourglass in which participants start off with their attention wide and receptive to any sounds that arrive to them, followed by a narrowing of their focus to their breath, which is then followed by a widening of their awareness inside their body (Figure S3.2).

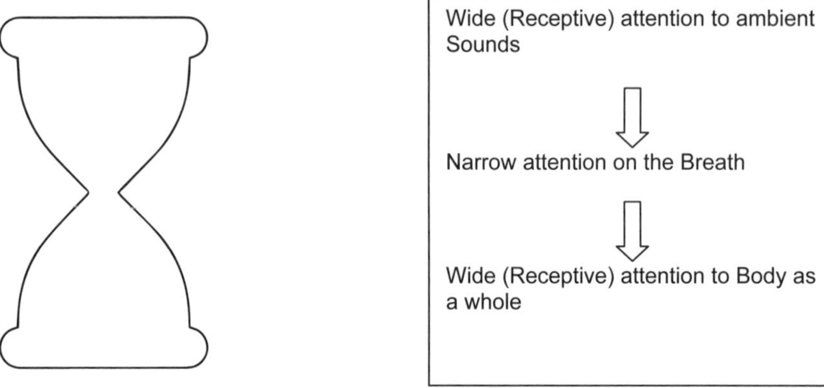

FIGURE S3.2. Hourglass meditation.

ADAPTATION TO INDIVIDUAL THERAPY

The Sound, Breath, and Body meditation can be practiced in two different ways. The first way, presented above, starts with receptive attention to ambient sounds, moving to a narrow attentional focus of the breath and ending with receptive attention to the body as a whole. The direction of awareness here is from the outside environment to the inside of the person and follows an hourglass analogy (similar to a 3-minute breathing space used in MBCT). The other way is to start with a narrow focus on the breath, move to the receptive focus of the whole body, and end with the receptive and wide focus on the ambient sounds. In individual therapy, both ways can be practiced and the patient is encouraged to reflect on what they notice and which way is easier for them.

The MT can introduce the practice in the following way:

"One way to curb daydreaming is to develop the habit of matching your attention with a previously set intention. You can do this by asking yourself: 'Where is my attention right now? Is my attention matching my intention?' This next exercise is about noticing your attention and shifting it if you notice it is breaking away from what you intended to focus on. This exercise will put you in the driver's seat of your attention and strengthen your ability to make transitions in your focus. If you notice your attention stray, ask yourself 'Where is my attention right now?' or 'Is my attention matching my intention?' "

SOUND, BREATH, AND BODY (EXERCISE 3.5)

[*Ring bell.*]

Find your meditation posture and take a few deeper breaths to relax before you begin.

First, we set the intention to notice sounds. Bring awareness to any sounds present, either within you or outside of you.

Receive the sounds by simply noting the coming and going of sounds without reaching for them.

Practice noticing sounds without creating a story about them, or judging or analyzing the sounds.

Whenever you catch yourself distracted or thinking during this exercise, silently label it as "thinking" or "daydreaming" and gently return to simply hearing sounds. [*Pause for 1–2 minutes*.]

Now, we shift and set the intention to notice your breath.

Let go of the sounds and bring attention to the sensations of your breathing in its natural flow.

Focus on the area where you feel the breath the most, and notice sensations as you take a breath in and sensations as you take a breath out. [*Pause for 1–2 minutes*.]

Now, we set the intention to notice any other body sensations that may be present.

Open attention to your whole body. You can notice your posture or sense your body weight resting on your seat.

Bring curiosity to your body and explore it from the inside, noting any feeling of pressure or tightness, itching or tingling, discomfort or pain, urge to move or general restlessness.

Notice if sensations are coming or going or notice if your attention is grabbed from one place to another. [*Pause for 1–2 minutes*.]

Now, let go of the body sensations and set the intention to be receptive to the present moment. Without a chosen object of attention, simply be aware of how your attention moves spontaneously from moment by moment. Practice being a witness of the awareness stream.

Whenever you catch yourself distracted or thinking, gently return to one of the three anchors of sound, breath, or body to again establish present moment awareness.

As we end, once again offer yourself some appreciation for sitting through this practice . . . learning to set intention, direct attention, and explore the flow of awareness.

I'm going to ring the bell in a moment. When I do, remember to listen to the bell's ring for its full duration. Once you no longer hear the bell, go ahead and open your eyes.

[*Ring bell*.]

After the exercise, the MT asks participants to share their experiences. If they are not spontaneously offered during the discussion, the MT also elicits answers on how this exercise can help with mind wandering. For participants who say it's difficult to focus on only one thing, the MT introduces the concept of foreground and background awareness. Some participants may think that they can either be focused or unfocused. The MT introduces that this is a false dichotomy: participants can be aware of something, but it may be part of the background awareness. With this description, the MT describes how some things can be in the foreground of their focus, while other things may be in the background of their focus. For example, they may be at work focused on a high-priority task, but they may also be aware of a background noise (e.g., coworkers having a conversation) that may tempt them to disengage from the high-priority task. As this applies to the formal mindfulness meditation exercises, participants may have an awareness of sounds in the foreground even when their awareness of their breathing is in the background. Once they want to make a switch to focus on the breath, they can shift the breath to the foreground and allow sounds to fall into the background. For some participants, it may be helpful to provide a visual depiction of what is meant by considering the foreground or background. Using Figure S3.3, the MT can explain how we can focus on the foreground, but there may be other items that are within awareness

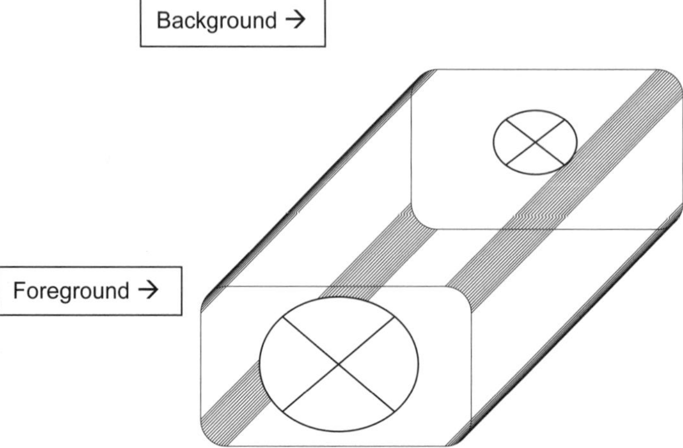

FIGURE S3.3. Items in our awareness can be in the foreground or the background at any moment.

as well, such as items in the background. Ask participants, "When your mind strays to those objects outside of the foreground, can you catch your mind wandering and ask yourself to come back to the foreground?"

S.T.O.P. INTRODUCTION AND PRACTICE

The MT introduces the S.T.O.P. exercise as another way to practice mindfulness in daily life:

S = Stop (or pause)
T = Take a breath and relax
O = Observe the present moment
P = Proceed

S.T.O.P. is presented as an all-purpose practice that can be used to mindfully observe the present moment. The MT encourages participants to use this brief practice to observe sounds, breath, and body—the three anchors—throughout the day. In later sessions, the S.T.O.P. practice can be expanded to also include observation of thoughts, feelings, and interactions (see Handout 3.1 for a summary).

S.T.O.P. PRACTICE (EXERCISE 3.6)

Sit comfortably and close your eyes.

[*Ring bell.*]

Today we will use the S.T.O.P. practice to bring mindful presence into moments of our lives.

In this practice, the letter *S* reminds us to stop, or pause, and let go of busy thinking or doing.

The letter *T* reminds us to take a few deeper breaths, anchoring attention on the sensations of the breath coming in and going out.

Next, the letter *O* reminds us to observe in the present moment. See if you can open your awareness to notice anything else that is here: any sounds, body sensations, thoughts, feelings, needs.

Observe the stream of experiences coming and going, noticing the shifts in your awareness and coming back to the breath as the anchor if you find yourself distracted or caught in thinking.

[*Pause.*]

As we end the meditation, the letter *P* reminds us we can proceed into the next moment now with more awareness.

[*Ring bell.*]

CLOSING

Discussion of Home Practice

The following at-home practice is discussed with the group. These are the basic points to convey (also summarized in Handout 3.2).

The formal practice is the 10-minute Mindfulness of Sound, Breath, and Body exercise daily. Ensure that participants have picked a time and place each day that is conducive with successfully meeting this goal. Consistent with the previous session, participants should track difficulties that emerge while engaging in the 10-minute formal mindfulness exercise each day. Track the formal practice using Handout 3.2.

There are two informal practice suggestions for this week:

1. Sound and walking or S.T.O.P. practice. Track using Handout 3.2 and refer to Handout 3.1 for a summary.
2. Use the attention check-in skill daily. With this skill, participants use visual cues as external reminders to ask themselves the following questions to regulate their attention: "Where is my attention right now?" and "What am I doing right now?" Explain to participants that this will help them get out of being in a state of mindlessness, like when we're on autopilot or daydreaming, by being more present in the moment with what they are doing.

BRIEF APPRECIATION MEDITATION (EXERCISE 3.7)

At the close of this session, introduce a short meditation lasting about 2 minutes that includes a moment to stop and reflect on the session just completed and appreciation for participants, including themselves. Invite participants to offer appreciation or loving-kindness to themselves for making the time to practice mindfulness and self-care, and offer appreciation to others for their presence in the class. The short closing meditation allows participants to experience positive emotions and gratefulness. Here's how the exercise might be narrated:

We close with a short appreciation practice. Sit in a relaxed yet upright posture and either close your eyes or keep them resting in one spot.

[*Ring bell.*]

Take a moment to appreciate everyone's presence today. People attending the group are here to care for themselves or to better their situations. The reasons may differ, but everyone is here to grow and improve their lives. Also, bring a sense of appreciation to yourself, for being here and taking the time for learning about yourself and mindfulness. See if you can connect with a sense of appreciation and gratitude in your body as you offer it to others and yourself.

[*Ring bell.*]

Depending on the amount of time left in the session, for a slightly longer version of this exercise that incorporates components of loving-kindness mindfulness meditation, you may want to incorporate the following into the exercise above:

In your mind, say the following to others: "May you be happy, may you be safe, may you be healthy and live with ease." *[Repeat this line two or three more times.]*

Avoid forcing a sense of appreciation. Instead, simply ask yourself if it's there already. If it's not there, just setting the intention to appreciate the presence of others is important.

Now, take a moment and offer yourself loving-kindness for making the time to practice mindfulness and take care of yourself, which will then help you take care of others and situations once you walk out of this room.

In your mind, say the following to yourself: "May I be happy, may I be safe, may I be healthy and live with ease." *[Repeat this line two or three more times.]*

Take this feeling of appreciation with you, but before you mentally leave the room, take this moment to sit and allow yourself to experience the positive emotion and a sense of gratefulness.

Let it spread in your body and move outward with you as you move on to the next part of your day.

[*Ring bell.*]

The weekly Home Practice Sheet (Handout 3.2) is given at the end of session. If the MT decides to send weekly email summaries after the group is completed, please refer to the end of Session 1 for an example of the structure of those emails. Also, see Session 1 for adaptation for individual therapy.

SESSION 4

Mindful Awareness of Body Sensations

SESSION SUMMARY

Overview

The theme of this session is the development of greater awareness of body sensations. Body awareness is fostered through a Body Scan exercise and developing ways to work mindfully with discomfort such as pain or restlessness. Mindful awareness of a daily activity is practiced through an informal exercise of putting on or taking off shoes. We find that people—even MTs new to the MAPs for ADHD Program—initially tend to be uncertain about how awareness of body sensations relates to ADHD. Therefore, we provide a rationale for this link in the theme introduction. Once participants are considering body sensations and how they are linked to their ADHD, they can approach situations involving problematic ADHD behaviors by either adopting a mind-body shift or practicing an acceptance-based perspective.

Session Outline

1) Brief opening meditation exercise: Sound, Breath, and Body (*Exercise 4.1*)
2) Review
    - Content of previous session
    - At-home practice experiences
3) Session theme: Being in the body
4) Body Scan (*Exercise 4.2*)
5) Break
6) Working with Pain and Discomfort (*Exercise 4.3*)

7) Mindfulness in daily life: Shoe Tying (*Exercise 4.4*)
8) Closing
   - Discussion of home practice
   - Brief Appreciation Meditation (*Exercise 4.5*)

Home Practice

1) Formal mindfulness practice: Sound, Breath, and Body (10 minutes per day)
2) Informal mindfulness practice:
   - Choosing a problematic ADHD-related activity (e.g., placement of keys)
   - Noticing your own ADHD symptoms with curiosity

BRIEF OPENING MEDITATION EXERCISE: SOUND, BREATH, AND BODY

This session starts with a brief meditation exercise that ties in an aspect of the practice learned last week. The opening practice also helps participants to quiet down, relax into the meeting, and become more present.

MINDFULNESS OF SOUND, BREATH, AND BODY (EXERCISE 4.1)

For this session's practice, we recommend awareness of the three anchors to the present moment discussed in the previous session: sound, breath, and body.

[*Ring bell.*]

In this practice, start by finding a comfortable sitting position. Keep your back straight yet relaxed as if you are sitting in a posture of dignity. Place your hands on your lap or by your side.

In this practice, we are becoming aware of the present moment using the anchors of sound, breath, and body. The three anchors are always here, always in the present.

First notice what sounds you hear. This does not mean looking for sounds, rather just being receptive to whatever sounds come and go, moment by moment, without judging or thinking about them. Simply hearing sounds as sounds, while avoiding making up stories about the sounds. The mind will bring up associations and judgments and yet we practice simply listening, simply receiving the sounds. You may ask yourself, "Are the sounds close to me or far away? Are they sounds within my body or outside of it? Is the sound prominent in the foreground or faint and in the background?" As you observe, notice the silences within and between sounds as well.

Now bring your attention to the breath. You can ask, "What is my breath like right now?" Simply be curious and notice the sensations of taking a breath in and out. You may also notice the pauses or moments of transitions between the in-breath and the out-breath.

Now shift your attention to other body sensations. What else do you notice in your body? Are there any sensations of tightness or looseness? Warmth or coolness? Do you notice your awareness shifting all over the body or going to one place in particular?

[*Ring bell.*]

REVIEW

Content of Previous Session

The MT discusses the formal and informal practices introduced in the previous session, as well as how the lesson related to ADHD. We recommend that MTs conduct this as a discussion and elicit feedback from participants who are "experts in their own ADHD." Therefore, while MTs are able to articulate how mindfulness practice from the previous week should map onto ADHD, participants should be able to comment on how this played out during their weekly practice. MTs should also encourage participants to use the handouts from the previous session to help them recall the major content and use of skills in the last week.

At-Home Practice Experiences

The following questions are asked to facilitate the review, starting with the informal practice (since informal practice may have been easier for participants to do during the week):

- "How many of you practiced mindfulness of sounds and walking in your informal exercise? For those who did, what did you notice?"
- "What was your experience with using the attention check-in? Did you practice asking yourself 'Where is my attention right now?' and 'What am I doing right now?'" As participants provide examples, ask them how they reminded themselves to ask themselves these questions and identify any practical behavioral strategies other participants may be able to adopt.
- "For your formal exercise, how was your experience with the sound, breath, and body meditation?"

As emphasized before, MTs discuss the above while balancing validation of any ongoing practice difficulties participants may have, with encouragement to persist. MTs should also observe the group process and keep reminding members to reflect on their own experiences versus providing advice to others. MTs can emphasize that such first-person sharing helps others tune into their own experience and share it with the group. While encouragement and validation of each other often arise spontaneously in the group process, and is a valuable aspect of the group experience, MTs should monitor the process and keep reminding participants to focus on sharing their own experiences.

ADAPTATION TO INDIVIDUAL THERAPY

The validating power of sharing that participants can provide each other is obviously not an option for those in individual therapy. The MT can choose to reflect on his or her own difficulties with mindfulness practice, to normalize the experience, while validating unique challenges of those with ADHD. It may also be helpful to connect the patient with a local ADHD support group or a general mindfulness meditation group in the area and reflect on such group experiences in the individual sessions.

SESSION THEME: BEING IN THE BODY

The main theme of this session is **being in the body**. This theme is related to learning how ADHD manifests in the body on a daily basis. The participants are taught to pay attention to their bodies in the formal and informal exercises that will be introduced in this session. The practices include focusing on physical sensations while sitting still as well as during body movements.

We recommend that MTs ask participants how ADHD may "show up in your body." Typically, we consider ADHD a disorder that involves impaired cognitive functioning (e.g., poor attention regulation and deficient executive functioning) or general restlessness and impulsivity. MTs encourage curiosity about body sensation, such as deeper, more specific awareness of how restlessness occurs and what happens in the body before or during impulsive actions. The following prompts and questions can be used:

- "Notice if there is any fidgetiness, and if so, where in your body is it located?"
- "Notice if it is hard for you to stay seated. How does that manifest in your body?"
- "If there is restlessness, what kind of movement would you like to do? What happens when you move? Does the feeling change when you move? What parts of your body typically communicate to you that you feel restless?"
- The MT can also introduce an example of impatience—difficulty waiting your turn, which is a common ADHD feature—and ask how that can show up in the body: "Where in your body do you feel the frustration or angst when you think you just can't wait anymore?"
- "Is there a body sensation right before you interrupt or do something impulsive?"
- "What do you notice about the effect your medications have on your symptoms and/or your body?"

These examples are not exhaustive but are exemplary for hyperactive-impulsive symptoms. Similarly, MTs may inquire about how inattentive ADHD symptoms manifest in the body, such as:

- "How does your body feel when you are ready to work on a task? How is it when you don't like the task? Does a thought of certain tasks change your body energy or state? What activities feel energizing or relaxing to your body? What brings on body tension?"
- "What do you notice in your body after you avoid, dislike, or are reluctant to do a task over a long period of time? Does your body begin to feel uncomfortable when you think about doing these things? Where in your body does this discomfort show up?"
- Among those who experience feeling overwhelmed when faced with a decision, complex situations, or difficult tasks, MTs may ask: "How does the overwhelmed feeling affect your breath and body?"

MTs may also discuss stress that results from ADHD symptoms, such as body tension that participants experience because they overcommitted because of poor planning or poor time management. The body sensation associated with stress may have been preceded by an ADHD behavior. Ask group members how noticing stress in the body may be a cue that their ADHD "is acting up."

More broadly, MTs may ask questions to group members about how attending to their body cues may be a way to reorient them toward their physical health. MTs might ask, "Can listening to your body help inform your physical well-being?"—suggesting that attending to body cues may provide an opportunity to change behavior. For example, group members who may overeat can be invited to ask themselves what the sensations of feeling full after a meal are like. When they notice those sensations using mindfulness, they create an opportunity to purposefully decide what to do next with the food in front of them. The increased awareness of body cues can also guide participants toward healthier lifestyle choices, such as noticing a spike in energy and then a crash after drinking a sugary beverage and ultimately deciding to limit such drinks from one's diet. In another example, MTs can discuss how stimulants can cause appetite suppression and encourage skipping meals, and how greater awareness of the body cues of fatigue, headache, or dehydration can prompt participants to better tend to their physical needs.

To emphasize some of the overall themes of this discussion, MTs may state something like, "One of the main points here is that the external distractions or busy ADHD mind often takes attention away from what your body is feeling. Yet your body may have a message for you, and we want to use mindfulness to help you stop and notice whenever your body has something to communicate. If you're not listening to your body, you may miss important information. Or you miss opportunities to regulate or shift your body state versus being driven by it. The goal is to focus on your body and learn how your ADHD or stress manifest in your body. This may not be easy at first, or it may feel uncomfortable, but as you practice tuning in, it will become easier to notice subtle shifts." Overall, MTs are encouraged to instruct participants to notice physical sensations that occur within their bodies with curiosity, without judgment or resistance, and with compassion using a phrasing similar to: "The body offers us messages—are you listening?"

The body offers us messages—are you listening?

In traditional mindfulness-based interventions like MBSR, this is typically the time when the difference between pain and suffering is discussed. While pain typically elicits thoughts of physical pain, this can also refer to psychological pain—participants with ADHD may be more likely to relate to the latter in terms of their presenting concerns that led to seeking treatment in the first place. Therefore, MTs may want to discuss how psychological pain correlates with discomfort. This can be discomfort that naturally arises for participants, such as feeling restless when they have to sit for long periods of time or feeling unfocused during a task they typically avoid. MTs teach that resistance to pain/discomfort can create suffering, and that pushing away pain/discomfort may create more suffering in life. In other words: "In life, pain is inevitable but suffering is optional."

We recommend that MTs discuss how pain/discomfort typically cannot be avoided and is part of our daily lives. For instance, sometimes distractibility or restlessness will emerge. One's relationship with this pain/discomfort will impact how it's experienced.

When participants practice radical acceptance of this pain/discomfort in a nonreactive way by adopting an attitude of openness, suffering can be reduced. MTs should try to elicit examples. Essentially this can be the difference between only getting distracted versus getting distracted plus being annoyed with yourself for getting distracted. Finally, MTs should also introduce how to work with pain/discomfort when it arises in the body. For example, instead of pushing away the experience of restlessness, gently leaning in toward the discomfort with a curiosity of what that experience is like.

BODY SCAN

The MT introduces a new mindfulness exercise: Body Scan. This guided formal mindfulness meditation exercise instructs participants to apply mindfulness to a very slow and deliberate "scanning" of various regions of the body and focusing their attention on the sensations there. A metaphor of a flashlight is used to help direct attention. The exercise involves moving attention slowly from head to toe as if "visiting and illuminating each part of the body." This exercise is typically done sitting in a chair, but may be done lying on the floor as well.

BODY SCAN (EXERCISE 4.2)

For this exercise, we will practice awareness of the sensations in our body. This is called a body scan. It is a great way to relax your body and bring more concentration and focus. With this exercise, we use our mindfulness to notice our body from head to toe.

First close your eyes, let your body relax, and get comfortable in your chair.

[*Ring bell.*]

Take a few deep breaths. Imagine that your attention is like a flashlight and you are pointing it and illuminating each part of your body. We start by bringing attention to the top of the head. See if you can notice any sensation there. A sensation is anything you feel in your body—it may be a very strong sensation or a very subtle one. The sensation may be pleasant, unpleasant, or neutral.

Maybe there are prickly or vibrating feelings, maybe it feels tingly or soft. Notice these in silence by simply paying attention and labeling them in your mind.

Anything you feel is fine. Also, you may not feel anything at all. Just be curious no matter what you notice.

Now, continuing from the top of your head, move your attention to your forehead and then your face. Pause and notice any sensations there.

As you scan your body, notice any feelings of impatience, wanting to rush, or other thoughts that arise. Label them, such as "impatience," then return to the scanning process. In this way, you are practicing patience.

Bring attention to your eyes—relax the area around your eyes. Move attention to your cheeks and then to your nose. Notice the area around your mouth and relax your jaw. Notice your chin. Now feel the back of your head and see if there are any sensations there. Or perhaps it is difficult to feel anything there. Finally notice your neck and throat and see whatever sensations are there.

Now swing your attention to your left shoulder and notice if there is anything to notice there.

You can also imagine that your attention is like a caring, soothing touch. Whenever you place your attention, let an intention of caring about yourself and your body infuse the area.

With your attention, feel your upper left arm, your elbow, and now your lower arm and hand. Then feel all five fingers.

Now move your attention to your right shoulder, feel your right upper arm, right elbow, lower arm, hand, and fingers.

Come back up to your back and scan your upper back for any sensations. You may not feel anything, or maybe you feel some discomfort or some pressure or tingles or itches.

Scan your attention across your back and down your spine to your lower back.

Now come up to your chest and feel sensations in your chest.

Notice your belly, including sensations of your breath there. Take your time, we don't have to rush here.

Notice how your body is sitting on the chair, noticing sensations around your hips and your buttocks and the seat.

Next bring attention to your left leg from the hip to the knee. Feel the knee and the calf. Notice sensations around your knee before moving toward the ankle. Feel the foot and all five toes.

Place your attention in your right hip and feel the right thigh, the knee, the calf, and then the ankle. Feel your foot and then your toes. When you reached the bottom, notice your whole body. Notice what it feels like now. *[Leave about 30 seconds of silence and then ring the bell.]*

The MT invites the participants to *share their experience with the above practice* and uses their comments to guide the discussion. During this discussion, the MT inquires if experiences that participants noticed during body scan are part of how ADHD typically manifests in daily life. Furthermore, the MT can inquire about how an enhanced awareness of body sensations—such as what participants just experienced—could impact how their ADHD is expressed in their daily lives.

BREAK

This is approximately the midpoint in the session, where a 5- to 10-minute break is taken.

WORKING WITH PAIN AND DISCOMFORT

We introduce this practice by inquiring with participants about any physical discomfort, such as pain or restlessness, that they may be experiencing currently. For a group of adults with ADHD, chronic pain complaints such as back pain or other forms of pain may not be as common as it may be in standard MBSR classes. Therefore, we also recommend inquiring about discomfort, such as restlessness, impatience, or inner tension that has some kind of physical component. In either case—whether focusing on pain or restlessness—the participants are led through a sequence of (1) noticing and describing the discomfort area (we will refer to "pain" here, but this can be used interchangeably with "restlessness") and (2) moving attention to a neutral body sensation (e.g., the breath or the palms of their hands). This back and forth between the discomfort and the neutral sensation is explored throughout the following silent practice. Instruct participants that they will work with discomfort using mindfulness techniques.

WORKING WITH PAIN AND DISCOMFORT (EXERCISE 4.3)

[*Ring bell.*]

Close your eyes and identify an area of your body in which you feel pain or discomfort. If you can't identify an area, think about those areas of your body where discomfort typically arises.

See if you can radically accept the pain or discomfort's presence. Can you open yourself up to its presence and let go of any agenda to fight or resist it? You don't have to like it—simply allow it to be there and don't automatically push it away with impatience. Instead, be curious about this experience. See if you can explore the pain as simply a sensation experienced by your body.

When you think about the pain or discomfort, see if you can describe it without personally identifying with it. For example, it's not "my pain," but a temporary sensation, such as "a sharp feeling." Instead of "I'm in pain," say "tingling" or whatever else is more descriptive of your experience without personalizing.

Let's explore the experience a bit more. What are the physical boundaries of the pain or discomfort? Is it localized to a certain area, such as the center of your forehead, or broadly distributed, such as all over your head?

Is the experience changing or remaining the same as this exercise progresses?

Do you notice any thoughts arising that may be judging the experience? Notice any thoughts as thoughts—no more than thoughts, no less than thoughts. They are events passing in your mind. Now, shift your attention to a neutral or comfortable spot, like your breath or the palms of your hands. Focus there for a bit and relax.

Again shift your attention back to the painful or uncomfortable area. After exploring the sensation a bit more, return to the neutral or comfortable spot, especially if the pain feels intense.

Move back and forth as needed from the area of your body where you feel pain or discomfort to the area of your body where you feel neutral or comfort. Notice how you're doing something different—coming back to the area you might typically avoid. Bring a sense of curiosity and ask yourself, "What can I learn from this experience that I might typically avoid?"

Bring an attitude of gentleness and compassion to yourself as you investigate the sensation.

[*Ring bell.*]

At the conclusion of this exercise, invite participants to share their experiences.

MTs may also want to consider incorporating Mindfulness of Movement or Mindfulness of Walking exercises (*Exercises 3.4* and *2.4,* respectively) into the practice above for participants who may prefer to move.

MINDFULNESS IN DAILY LIFE: SHOE TYING

To add to the discussion about physical sensations and ADHD, MTs can revisit the theme from Session 1 about being in "automatic pilot" mode and contrast this with mindful awareness. To exemplify, MTs can discuss patterns of losing focus or spacing out, multitasking, failing to finish tasks, being forgetful, and losing things as examples of being in automatic pilot mode. While participants will ultimately want to bring a mindful awareness to these behaviors since they likely led participants to seek out this treatment, we typically start with the more benign behavior of shoe tying, which doesn't carry all of the self-critical internal dialogue that participants might have when they catch themselves engaging in ADHD behaviors.

The MT can introduce the mindful shoe-tying exercise in the following way:

> "Today we are going to do to practice being mindful of something we do every day but often don't pay attention to. We're going to mindfully take our shoes on and off. When you put on your shoes, what are you usually thinking about? [*Take answers.*] Right, usually we are thinking about all sorts of things, but not our shoes. Why? Because putting on shoes is a habit. When we do activities that are habits, we usually space out and are not mindful.
>
> "What other activities do you typically 'space out' while doing? [*Take answers.*]
>
> "During things like brushing teeth, doing our chores, getting dressed, all of these things, because they are habits, we are not mindful. So let's learn to be mindful when we do a daily activity or habit."

SHOE TYING (EXERCISE 4.4)

We are going to do this activity in slow motion with enhanced present-moment awareness. Move as slowly as you possibly can while paying attention to the moment-by-moment changes in your experience. We will do this silently, not talking or making other noises. Please pay attention carefully to the instructions so you don't get ahead of the class.

Everyone bend down to untie, unbuckle, or un-Velcro one shoe. If there's nothing to undo, you can still bend down. As you do it, notice your body sensations. Notice your torso moving, notice your arm reaching out, feel the sensations. Slow down if you find yourself rushing through the motions.

Now reach for the tie or buckle if you have one. Put all your attention in the feeling in your fingers. Slowly untie the bow or unbuckle your shoe, noticing what you feel.

Then move your hands to take the shoe off slowly. Notice if there is heat or coolness or relief in the foot. Now wiggle your toes. Notice how your foot feels. Tense? Loose? Great.

Now in silence, very slowly, without me talking, put your shoe back on. Continue to be mindful of the movement and sensations as you do it.

[*Give remainder of the time in silence and ring the meditation bell at end.*]

At the end of this exercise, MTs ask participants about their experience. Prompts to get the discussion going might be:

- "How do you normally take off your shoes?"
- "Why was it different today? Did you notice anything about this mundane act that you haven't noticed before?"
- "Could you imagine doing this every time you take off your shoes?"

MTs remind participants that they can practice mindfulness any time they put on or take off their shoes. As the discussion progresses, MTs can ask participants to consider other activities for which they could practice mindfulness in very slow motion. At this point, suggestions might be more relevant to ADHD. For example, for participants who say they are frequently forgetful about where they place their keys, how could practicing being mindfully aware and progressing through this behavior very slowly and with enhanced awareness change this behavior? For topics that arise that MTs can demonstrate in session, such as forgetfulness, this is an opportunity to repeat the exercise above. If we stick with the example of being forgetful about the placement of keys, the MT asks participants to take their keys out and notice the physical sensation of the keys in their hand (e.g., do they feel warm or cool?). The following prompts can be used: "Can you visually inspect the keys? Can you set down the keys with a visual awareness of how they settle onto the table and an auditory awareness of the sound they make?" After this discussion and impromptu exercise, the MT discusses how this practice can help ADHD behaviors. It is helpful to point out that by slowing down with enhanced sensory awareness of the activity, we have more information to encode. Thus, slow, mindful awareness of key placement can later help with recall of where the keys were placed.

Participants may mention how moving slowly and mindfully through tasks that they otherwise do on automatic pilot will be difficult because of the time and cognitive effort it takes. MTs can acknowledge that this is one of the benefits of being in automatic pilot mode and that this is an adaptive process. For instance, it is preferable to put on your own shoes without thinking about the nuances of that behavior, such as how to tie shoelaces. However, we are focusing this approach for the times when being in automatic pilot mode corresponds with ADHD behaviors that cause problems. In those situations, a gentle reminder to "go slow" will initially take effort for participants, but this will become easier as they continue to practice.

CLOSING

Discussion of Home Practice

The following at-home practice is discussed with the group. These are the basic points to convey (also summarized in Handout 4.1).

The formal practice is the 10-minute Mindfulness of Sound, Breath, and Body exercise or Body Scan daily. Ensure that participants have picked a time and place each day that is conducive to successfully meeting this goal.

There are two informal practices for this week:

1. Choose a problematic ADHD-related activity that involves the body (e.g., placement of keys or wallet) and practice mindfulness of physical sensations in daily life in a way that is similar to Exercise 4.4. For participants who struggle to identify an activity, they can practice taking on and off their shoes.
2. Consistent with previous sessions, observe your own ADHD symptoms with curiosity in daily life. Optional Handout 2.3 can be used or participants may wish to use their own journal to write about their ADHD. Whatever the medium for mindfully observing one's own ADHD, follow this session's emphasis on body sensations.

BRIEF APPRECIATION MEDITATION (EXERCISE 4.5)

At the close of this session, introduce a short meditation lasting about 2 minutes that includes a moment for participants to stop and reflect on the session just completed and appreciation for all participants, including themselves. Invite participants to offer appreciation or loving-kindness to themselves for making the time to practice mindfulness and self-care, and offer appreciation to others for their presence in the class. The short closing meditation allows participants to experience positive emotions and gratefulness. Here's how the exercise might be narrated:

> We close with a short appreciation practice. Sit in a relaxed yet upright posture and either close your eyes or keep them resting in one spot.
>
> [*Ring bell.*]
>
> Take a moment to appreciate everyone's presence today. People attending the group are here to care for themselves or to better their situations. The reasons may differ, but everyone is here to grow and improve their lives. Also, bring a sense of appreciation to yourself, for being here and taking the time for learning about yourself and mindfulness. See if you can connect with a sense of appreciation and gratitude in your body as you offer it to others and yourself.
>
> [*Ring bell.*]

Depending on factors like amount of time left in the session, for a slightly longer version of this exercise that incorporates components of loving-kindness mindfulness meditation, you may want to incorporate the following into the exercise above:

> In your mind, say the following to others: "May you be happy, may you be safe, may you be healthy and live with ease." [*Repeat this line two or three more times.*]
>
> Avoid forcing a sense of appreciation. Instead, simply ask yourself if it's there already. If it's not there, just setting the intention to appreciate the presence of others is important.
>
> Now, take a moment and offer yourself loving-kindness for making the time to practice mindfulness and take care of yourself, which will then help you take care of others and situations once you walk out of this room.
>
> In your mind, say the following to yourself: "May I be happy, may I be safe, may I be healthy and live with ease." [*Repeat this line two or three more times.*]
>
> Take this feeling of appreciation with you, but before you mentally leave the room, take this moment to sit and allow yourself to experience the positive emotion and a sense of gratefulness.
>
> Let it spread in your body and move outward with you as you move on to the next part of your day.
>
> [*Ring bell.*]

The weekly Home Practice Sheet (Handout 4.1) is given at the end of session. If MTs decide to send weekly email summaries after the group is completed, please refer to the end of Session 1 for an example of the structure of those emails. Also see Session 1 for adaptation for individual therapy.

SESSION 5

Mindful Awareness of Thoughts

SESSION SUMMARY

Overview

The theme of this session is the development of greater awareness of thoughts. Mindful awareness of thoughts is introduced by using a picture of the sky and clouds to demonstrate the difference between meta-awareness (represented as the blue sky) and present moment experiences (represented by clouds that can be different sensations, such as thoughts, feelings, mental images, sounds, or body sensations). Because many adults with ADHD, especially those with elevated hyperactive-impulsive symptoms, report restlessness in the body and in the mind, MTs can suggest that the active mind with the numerous thoughts it generates provides many opportunities to practice mindful awareness (or meta-awareness) of thinking and its patterns. In clinical practice and in research, adults with ADHD often report engaging in negativistic, overly critical, depressive thinking. At the same time, overly positive or optimistic thoughts are also common among adults with ADHD and can be maladaptive. The MTs can explore with the participants the functional impact of these exaggerated or out-of-balance thinking styles. Participants learn how nonjudgmental awareness is a step in the process of learning how to learn discernment and intentionally choosing more mindful actions. For the at-home practice, participants are asked to track their maladaptive cognitions and begin applying mindfulness to modify how they respond to these thoughts.

Session Outline

1) Brief opening meditation exercise: Body Scan (*Exercise 5.1*)
2) Review
    - Content of previous session
    - At-home practice experiences

3) Session theme: Mindful awareness of thoughts
4) Mindfulness of Thoughts (*Exercise 5.2*)
5) Break
6) Walking with Your Thoughts (*Exercise 5.3*)
7) ADHD and judgmental thoughts
8) Sharing Experiences with Judgmental Thoughts (*Exercise 5.4*)
9) Other out-of-balance thinking
10) Self-talk as a guide
11) Closing
    - Discussion of home practice
    - Brief Appreciation Meditation (*Exercise 5.5*)

Home Practice

1) Formal mindfulness practice: Mindfulness of Thoughts (10 minutes per day)
2) Informal mindfulness practice:
    - Daily tracking of judgmental thoughts
    - Noticing your own ADHD symptoms with curiosity

BRIEF OPENING MEDITATION EXERCISE: BODY SCAN

The MT starts with a brief meditation exercise that incorporates an aspect of the practice learned in the previous session. As in other sessions, this opening practice helps participants to quiet down, relax into the meeting, and become more present.

BODY SCAN (5 MINUTES) (EXERCISE 5.1)

For this session's practice, we recommend a short version of the Body Scan exercise.

[*Ring bell.*]

Start by finding a comfortable sitting position. Keep your back straight yet relaxed as if you are sitting in a posture of dignity. Place your hands on your lap or by your side.

In this practice, we become more aware of the body and bring attention to different body sensations. As you tune into your body, ask, "What is my body feeling like right now?"

Are there any sensations of tightness or looseness? Warmth or coolness? Do you notice your awareness shifting all over the body or going to one place in particular? Maybe there are prickly or vibrating feelings, maybe it feels tingly or soft. Whatever you notice, even if absence of sensation, it is okay. Notice your body in silence by simply paying attention to any sensations present and labeling them in your mind.

What part or parts of your body are you aware of right now? Anything you feel is fine. Also, you may not feel anything at all. Just be curious no matter what you notice.

Bring attention to the upper part of your body. Scan from the top of your head, down to your forehead, and your face, including your eyes, your cheeks, and your nose.

[*Pause.*]

Then move down further checking in with your neck, left shoulder, right shoulder, left elbow, right elbow, the tips of your fingers.

[*Pause.*]

Now notice your back from the top all the way down to your waist. What are you noticing? Finally scan both of your legs from your hips to your toes and notice the contact with the floor.

Breathe into these sensations and rest in the present moment.

[*Leave about 30 seconds of silence and then ring bell.*]

REVIEW

Content of Previous Session

The MT discusses the formal Body Scan exercise and informal practices from the previous session and relates them to ADHD: being in the body and learning how ADHD manifests in the body. The MT also reviews how to work through pain and discomfort with mindfulness. MTs should encourage participants to use the handouts from the previous session to help them recall the major content and use of skills in the last week.

At-Home Practice Experiences

The following questions are asked to facilitate the review, starting with the informal practice (since informal practice may have been easier for participants to do during the week):

- "How many of you practiced the Shoe Tying exercise or mindfully slowing down another activity? For those who did, how did it go and what did you notice?"
- "Our formal meditation exercises are now at 10 minutes. How did you do with your gradual increase in time spent meditating each day? Are there any 'tricks' you learned that might help others establish this new routine?"
- "What were any challenges that emerged from the Body Scan exercise? What were things you liked about the Body Scan exercise?"
- "Taking a look at the big picture for you, have you noticed anything about how the mindfulness meditation practices and lessons behind them are beginning to impact your ADHD or your life in general?"

MTs discuss the above with a balance of validation of any ongoing practice difficulties and encouragement to "stick with it."

ADAPTATION TO INDIVIDUAL THERAPY

In the individual therapy setting, MTs have greater flexibility to focus on unique challenges that are arising during the at-home practice. Whereas the group therapy setting does not allow for such in-depth focus on the individual, MTs may want to devote more time to difficulties patients are having implementing formal and informal practices. We recommend that MTs be prepared to integrate components of CBT for adults with ADHD so that they can support their patients' mindfulness practice, such as problem solving or stimulus control techniques. Compatibility issues in how cognitions are addressed in both MAPs and CBT are considered later on in this session.

SESSION THEME: MINDFUL AWARENESS OF THOUGHTS

The main theme of this session is **being more aware of one's own thoughts** on a daily basis and learning a meta-awareness stance when observing thinking. A picture of a sky and clouds (Figure S5.1) can be used as a visual aid to discuss how thoughts (depicted by clouds in the sky) are passing, temporary mental phenomena that can be noticed without overly identifying with them. The MT can reference this with the saying "You are not your thoughts." Participants are encouraged to observe "the passing thought clouds" and label or name them silently in their mind as a way to help de-identify from them: "Oh, there is a memory . . . a judgment . . . a worry," etc. The blue sky here represents awareness and a metacognitive stance: the participants are encouraged to realize that they can observe their thoughts and other mental experiences and yet be separate or "more than" such experiences. MTs can also point out that in the figure the passing mental experiences include thoughts as well as feelings, body sensations, images, sounds, and other experiences.

The MT emphasizes how the main skill learned at this point is to learn how to observe one's own mind and develop a different relationship with thoughts. Whereas traditionally participants may overly identify with and personalize their thoughts, in the MAPs for ADHD Program, they are encouraged to witness their thoughts as changing, impermanent phenomena that do not necessary represent the true reality. The MT

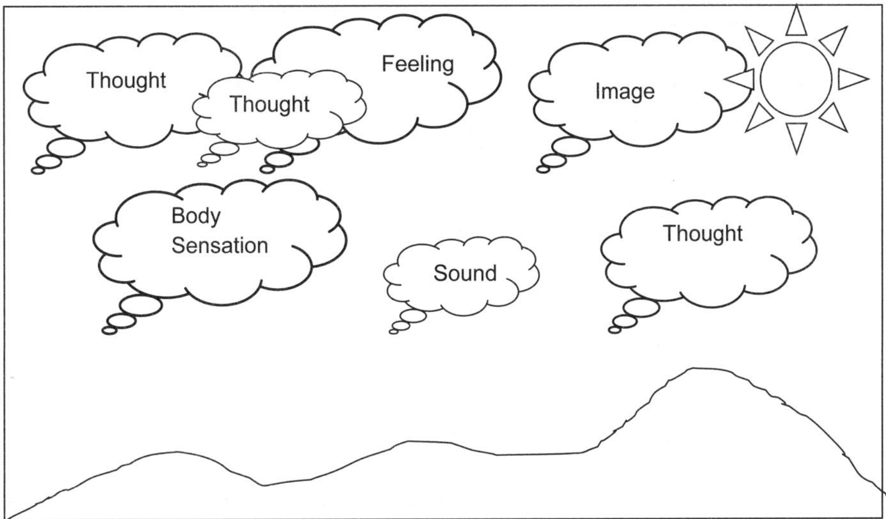

FIGURE S5.1. Illustration for discussion of the Mind Like a Sky concept.

can introduce the slogans or sayings: "You are not your thoughts" and "Don't believe everything you think" as quick reminders of the meta-cognitive stance this session is teaching. MTs should be aware that at this point in the session, cognitions commonly associated with their ADHD have not yet been addressed. We get to that later into the session, but for now the focus is on introducing a mindful view toward all mental phenomena using the formal mindfulness exercise below.

As a side note, although not discussed with the participants, MTs should think conceptually about how a mindfulness approach to cognitions might differ from a traditional CBT approach to cognitions. In traditional CBT, there is an emphasis on changing the content of thoughts and labeling thoughts as cognitive errors: "negative," "distorted," "irrational," or "erroneous." Traditional CBT encourages individuals to consider alternative ways to think about a given situation. In contrast, mindfulness-based intervention approaches, including the MAPs for ADHD Program, emphasize changing one's relationship with one's thoughts and viewing thoughts as private and impermanent mental phenomenon. Therefore, whereas in traditional CBT we may ask participants to engage with and change the content of cognitions, mindfulness-based interventions ask participants to witness the cognitions from a new stance without directly changing the content.[1]

We think that this alternative to a traditional CBT approach may be particularly suited for adults with ADHD given their cognitive style that can generate both overly negative and overly positive thoughts. That is, in addition to adults with ADHD often endorsing depressive cognitions (e.g., Mitchell at al., 2013), they also endorse overly positive or optimistic cognitions (Knouse, Mitchell, Kimbrel, & Anastopoulos, 2019; see Knouse & Mitchell, 2015, for a review). The latter might be typified by "I'm really good at doing things at the last minute," which is positive and viewed by participants as a strength, but is also likely maladaptive because in many cases it will lead to more procrastination, which is typical of adults with ADHD. When a traditional CBT approach is adopted, participants may or may not feel supported by their therapist when they receive feedback that their tendency to "think positive" is "distorted" or "irrational." Instead, a mindfulness approach sidesteps this potential reaction and allows MTs to address these cognitions (i.e., lower the cognitions' validity to the patients) without using the framing that may be perceived as negative in traditional CBT. Noting, letting go of the thoughts (without engaging in the content), then redirecting attention offers a helpful cognitive self-regulation strategy for those with ADHD.

MINDFULNESS OF THOUGHTS

The MT will introduce a new exercise: Mindfulness of Thoughts. As with many other formal practices, this exercise is typically practiced sitting in a chair, but may be done lying on the floor as well. For participants who want to move, Exercise 5.3, Walking with Your Thoughts, offers an alternative way of practicing.

---

[1] As opposed to *traditional* CBT approaches, more recent iterations of CBT in the past few years often incorporate a "third-generation" (see Chapter 2) approach to cognitions that is more aligned with the MAPs for ADHD Program. For an example of a CBT for adult ADHD that incorporates this "third generation" approach, see Ramsay (2020).

MINDFULNESS OF THOUGHTS (EXERCISE 5.2)

For this exercise, we will practice awareness of the thoughts going through your mind. This is called a mindfulness of thoughts exercise. With this exercise, we watch our thoughts without getting caught up in them.

First close your eyes, let your body relax and get comfortable in your chair.

[*Ring bell.*]

In this practice, you are invited to witness the flow of your thinking. Instead of getting caught up in your thoughts—which is all too easy to do—you are invited to practice observing your thinking as clouds floating across the sky.[2]

We start by becoming grounded in the present moment. Notice your breathing and allow yourself to relax in the here and now.

When your attention is relatively stable on the breath, open your awareness to thoughts you are having right now. Let the breath fall into the background and see if you can watch your thoughts float into and out of your awareness.

It may help to picture your mindful awareness as a spacious blue sky with clouds floating across it. Your awareness is like a big blue sky: vast and spacious, larger than the passing clouds. With this spacious awareness, you can watch your thoughts, feelings, and sensations as if they are clouds coming and going.

Check in with yourself and see if you can label any inner experiences without personalizing them. For example, "there's worry" or "a judgmental thought" or "a planning thought," "an image," or "a feeling."

Ask yourself, "Can I treat these thoughts for what they are: 'mental events'—no more, no less?"

Notice if your thoughts, like clouds, may move quickly or slowly. Maybe some thoughts are linked and tell a story, and some may be separate from one another. Are some of the thoughts light and fluffy clouds, or foreboding dark and heavy clouds?

Note the content and the impact that these thoughts have on you while, if possible, not being drawn into thinking about them. Instead of trying to grab for the thought and think through it, see if you can allow the thought to float by.

When you do this practice, it is easy to get lost in thinking. You may notice suddenly that you're enveloped by the cloud of thought. Whenever that occurs, shift your awareness to your breath and ground yourself in the present moment. Then, when you're ready, return to watching your thoughts.

Be curious if you can notice the space between you and your thoughts—the space is meta-awareness. This is a space where you can observe your mind without getting pulled by it. It is the space from which you can note thoughts and feelings, but choose not to act on them. I'm going to pause for a minute as you continue to observe your thoughts. *[Pause.]*

Note that an individual thought eventually goes away, even the ones that may feel like they'll last forever. Watching our thoughts helps us realize that they are impermanent. They come and go. See if you can notice this for yourself.

Note how some thoughts keep coming back. Maybe some thoughts are "I," "me," or "mine" thoughts. Can you, as the nonjudging observer or witness, let go of identifying with these thoughts and see them as "just thoughts"?

---

[2]If they are more familiar with alternative imagery to convey the same point, MTs can chose to use other metaphors in this practice. For example, thoughts can be described as leaves floating on a stream instead of clouds in the sky.

Observe any feelings and moods as they come and go along with the thoughts. Is there any aversion or disliking of some thoughts? Are there thoughts that are particularly pleasant and hard to let go of?

Remember to shift back to your breath if you get lost in thought.

We'll end this exercise by extending appreciation to yourself for pausing and noticing your thoughts from a new perspective.

[*Leave about 30 seconds of silence and then ring bell.*]

The MT invites the participants to share their experience with the above practice and uses their comments to guide the discussion. During this discussion, the MT inquires if experiences noticed during Mindfulness of Thoughts are part of how ADHD typically manifests in daily life. The MT encourages participants to reflect on how enhanced awareness of thoughts could impact how their ADHD is expressed in daily situations and their response to it.

ADAPTATION TO INDIVIDUAL THERAPY

After this practice, have patients draw a picture of a sky and write out the thoughts that emerged on their clouds. This can help patients further process these thoughts. This adaptation can also be carried out in group if time permits.

BREAK

This is approximately the midpoint in the session, where a 5- to 10-minute break is taken.

WALKING WITH YOUR THOUGHTS

For the next exercise, participants are guided through a short walking meditation focused on the sensations of the feet and legs while adding the new component of mindful awareness of thoughts. During this exercise, participants build on the walking exercise introduced in Session 2 (i.e., focusing on the sensations in their feet and legs as an attentional anchor while walking), then expand and shift their awareness to thinking. This further emphasizes the meta-awareness perspective in which participants are noticing thoughts with some distance from them, like watching clouds float by in the sky as they stand on the ground beneath. Whenever participants catch themselves getting lost in thought, they can bring their attention back to their feet or legs as an attentional anchor before returning back to observing their thoughts.

WALKING WITH YOUR THOUGHTS (EXERCISE 5.3)

For this exercise, we're going to slowly walk around the room in a large circle. Leave enough space between you and your neighbor. Since we'll be walking, we'll keep our eyes open. However, keep your eyes focused on what is immediately in front of you as you walk so that you minimize what is in your visual field that may otherwise distract you.

[*Ring bell.*]

Start off by slowly walking while attending to the lifting and falling of your legs. Notice how your feet meet and depart from the floor.

When your attention is relatively stable and anchored to the sensations at your feet, practice opening your awareness to your thinking. Your thoughts come into and leave your awareness, like clouds in the sky.

Practice perceiving your thoughts as "events" in your mind, noticing how they change moment by moment.

See if you can notice your thoughts without being lost in them, thinking about your thinking, or being drawn into the story in your mind. Instead, practice staying centered in the present moment and observing the process of thought.

See if you can keep your thoughts in the foreground of your attention while at the same time maintaining some awareness of the physical sensation of walking in the background.

Observing your thinking in this mindful way is not easy—simply try your best and be kind to yourself. If you get caught up in some kind of story, gently bring your attention back to your feet. Once you anchor your awareness, come back to noticing your thoughts.

[*Leave about 3 minutes of silence and then ring bell.*]

The MT debriefs with the participants and inquires how the walking practice differed for them from a sitting practice. The MT offers that each person can decide each day whether to do a sitting or a walking formal practice.

ADHD AND JUDGMENTAL THOUGHTS

The MT asks participants about their experience with judgmental, or overly harsh or critical, thoughts and how those thoughts relate to their ADHD. MTs may introduce how research has demonstrated that depressive, anxious, and perfectionistic cognitions that are deeply steeped in judgment are common among adults with ADHD (Abramovitch & Schweiger, 2009; Knouse, Zvorsky, & Safren, 2013; Mitchell et al., 2013; Strohmeier, Rosenfield, DiTomasso, & Ramsay, 2016). During this discussion, ask participants about the impact of these judgmental thoughts. Typically, this involves a discussion about self-esteem and how judgmental thoughts are quite painful or demotivating to participants.

Discuss how the MAPs for ADHD Program is focused on recognizing judgmental thoughts and how those thoughts can lead to amplifying problems that are common in ADHD.

SHARING EXPERIENCES WITH JUDGMENTAL THOUGHTS (EXERCISE 5.4)

Participants are asked to share about judgmental thoughts they tend to have. The sharing can be done in pairs or as a group. The MT provides prompts, such as:

- "How do judgmental thoughts toward yourself or others show up in your daily life currently? What about in the past?"
- "Do you judge yourself for being judgmental?"

MT should teach that mindfulness provides a way to neutralize judgmental thinking by noticing such thoughts without identifying with them and by observing how they affect things like the breath, the body, and mood. To help participants get these conversations started, the MT can start by providing some examples that may be more relevant for ADHD. MTs are encouraged to bring in examples from their own experience working with ADHD patients, though we provide some examples for guidance:

- "I've got the attention span of a gnat."
- "I'm not dependable—people who know me well know I will just flake out."
- "I am so stupid." (Or alternatively, "You are so stupid, how come you don't get what I am saying?")
- "Something is wrong with me."
- "People are so slow!"
- "This guy is a jerk!"
- "I just can't get my life together."
- "I'm such an idiot for getting distracted by things that others can ignore!"

Before starting this exercise, the MT reminds participants that as in any group therapy, it is important to be receptive, nonjudgmental, and kind toward other participants when they share their thoughts. Participants may already be reticent to share their judgmental thoughts out loud with other people. The title of a popular, classic ADHD book, *You Mean I'm Not Lazy, Stupid or Crazy?!* (Kelly & Ramundo, 2006), can be referenced as a common negative self-judgment in ADHD. As opposed to asking whether these judgments are right or wrong, or good or bad, MTs help participants reorient to the function of these judgments—do they have a negative impact? If so, the first step in de-identifying with such judgments to diffuse their impact is to simply note their presence. The MT can also reference a story of Coach A and Coach B (see the Adaptation to Individual Therapy box below).

ADAPTATION TO INDIVIDUAL THERAPY

We recommend adopting a story of Coach A and Coach B from other ADHD treatments (Safren, Perlman, Sprich, & Otto, 2005) and earlier iterations of this treatment (Zylowska, 2012) to demonstrate the positive effect adaptive self-talk can have on patients, which we summarize here. While we recommend considering this story in individual therapy, it can easily be incorporated into discussion in the group setting as well. This story helps patients to see how practicing self-compassion—a core feature of mindfulness—can be helpful when they experience judgmental thoughts toward themselves. Here's how the MT may want to introduce the story:

> "Imagine a little girl who is learning how to play baseball. In this example, let's call her Jenny. Jenny's learning how to catch a fly ball. Her coach hits one out to her, and she misses it despite her best effort. Coach A starts yelling, 'You should have caught that! You obviously weren't paying attention earlier—you can't do anything right! If you miss any more balls, I'm going to make you sit on the bench!'

"Now, how do you think Jenny feels? [*Allow time for your patient to respond and make sure you touch on feelings like less confidence, tension, and overwhelmed.*] Do you think she's going to be more or less likely to catch the next fly ball that comes toward her? [*Allow your patient time to respond.*] If anything, she's probably less likely to catch the ball. She's discouraged, and she didn't receive any corrective feedback to fix any errors she may be making.

"Let's go through the same scenario with Jenny, but this time Coach B says something without yelling at Jenny. Coach B says, 'Well, you missed that one and that's okay—you're learning. Here's what I want you to do next time: fly balls are tricky and you usually want to take a few steps backward when you first see it in the air, then run forward if you need to as it gets closer.'

"Now, how does Jenny feel after Coach B? Better than after Coach A, right? [*Allow time for your patient to respond and touch on feelings like greater confidence and feeling supported.*] Do you think she has a better shot at catching the next fly ball when you contrast Coach B with Coach A? [*Elicit from your patient how Jenny is probably not going to feel so overwhelmed that she'll want to quit and that maybe she's going to enjoy the game more.*]

OTHER OUT-OF-BALANCE THINKING

In addition to negative or judgmental thinking, research on cognitive styles among adults with ADHD has also demonstrated that overly positive cognitions are common as well (e.g., "I do better waiting until the last minute"; Knouse et al., 2019). Another example is thinking right before one should be leaving for an appointment: "I can still gather my laundry before I have to go," and consequently being late for the appointment. Explain to participants how both patterns of thinking—overly negative and overly positive—are common and can co-occur in the same person. Focus on the functional impact of these cognitions, such as avoidance of a cognitively demanding task until the last minute. This is also a good time to bring up how ADHD often comes with errors in assessment of time, leading to "overly optimistic" assumptions (or underestimation) of how long things take.

SELF-TALK AS A GUIDE

Consistent with the acceptance and change perspective, the MT introduces the concept of mindful self-talk or self-coaching. The MT discusses adopting a mindful approach toward one's current self-talk or self-narrative about one's behavior. The MT asks participants if they can invite self-talk that embraces some of the tenets of mindfulness (letting go of judgment, openness, curiosity, and compassion) when observing their behavior. Such mindful witnessing of thoughts and behavior (acceptance) is discussed as a necessary step in creating a new way of being and willingness to engage in values-oriented behavior (change). For example, the MT can ask participants, "Can your inner voice be used to stress the importance of being fully present and accepting of what's going on for you in a nonjudgmental, kind, and curious way?" For many participants with ADHD, procrastination is a typical problem. For that, the MT may want to ask participants to think about tasks they typically want to avoid and use their self-talk to guide them to (1) fully and nonjudgmentally acknowledge the procrastination and (2) engage in that task, even when they have a strong urge to put it off. For example, MTs might say, "Can this inner voice guide your next actions in a desired, valued direction—even if it's something you may not want to do right now?" The MT is asking participants both to accept urges to put off tasks and to change how they might respond to those urges.

CLOSING

Discussion of Home Practice

The MT should make sure to take sufficient time to review the plan for exercises to complete at home. This time is used to address questions, clarify any points of confusion, and "fill in the blanks" for any participants who may have experienced mind wandering during parts of the session or those who feel unsure about what is being asked of them in the week ahead. The following are the basic points to convey (also summarized in Handout 5.1).

The formal practice is the 10-minute Mindfulness of Thoughts exercise (i.e., Mind Like a Sky or Walking with Your Thoughts exercise) daily. Ensure that participants have chosen a time and place each day that is conducive to successfully meeting this goal, as well as a narrative to walk them through the exercise. They can track their progress using Handout 5.1.

There are two informal practices for this week:

1. Track judgmental thoughts that emerge over the next week. This can be accomplished in different ways, including during formal exercises or in everyday life. For example, participants can for one day count the frequency of judgmental thoughts and identify the content of these thoughts. Prompt participants to think about how they will keep track of what they observe. Handout 5.1 can be used for this.
2. Consistent with previous sessions, ask participants to observe their own ADHD symptoms with curiosity in daily life. Some participants may wish to use something other than the handout provided in the session. For example, participants may wish to create journal entries and provide more context about their ADHD. The medium for documenting this practice is less important than them gaining the knowledge about how ADHD plays out for them on a day-to-day basis, while also incorporating this session's emphasis on mindful awareness of thoughts. Optional Handout 2.3 may be used for this.

BRIEF APPRECIATION MEDITATION (EXERCISE 5.5)

At the close of this session, introduce a short meditation lasting about 2 minutes that includes a moment to stop and reflect on the session just completed and appreciation for participants, including themselves. Invite participants to offer appreciation or loving-kindness to themselves for making the time to practice mindfulness and self-care, and offer appreciation to others for their presence in the class. The short closing meditation allows participants to experience positive emotions and gratefulness. Here's how the exercise might be narrated:

> We close with a short appreciation practice. Sit in a relaxed yet upright posture and either close your eyes or keep them resting in one spot.
>
> [*Ring bell.*]
>
> Take a moment to appreciate everyone's presence today. People attending the group are here to care for themselves or to better their situations. The reasons may differ, but everyone is here to grow and improve their lives. Also, bring a sense of appreciation to yourself, for being here and taking the time for learning about yourself and mindfulness. See if you can connect with a sense of appreciation and gratitude in your body as you offer it to others and yourself.
>
> [*Ring bell.*]

Depending on factors like the amount of time left in the session, for a slightly longer version of this exercise that incorporates components of loving-kindness mindfulness meditation, you may want to incorporate the following into the exercise above:

> In your mind, say the following to others: "May you be happy, may you be safe, may you be healthy and live with ease." [*Repeat this line two or three more times.*]
>
> Avoid forcing a sense of appreciation. Instead, simply ask yourself if it's there already. If it's not there, just setting the intention to appreciate the presence of others is important.
>
> Now, take a moment and offer yourself loving-kindness for making the time to practice mindfulness and take care of yourself, which will then help you take care of others and situations once you walk out of this room.
>
> In your mind, say the following to yourself: "May I be happy, may I be safe, may I be healthy and live with ease." [*Repeat this line two or three more times.*]
>
> Take this feeling of appreciation with you, but before you mentally leave the room, take this moment to sit and allow yourself to experience the positive emotion and a sense of gratefulness.
>
> Let it spread in your body and move outward with you as you move on to the next part of your day.
>
> [*Ring bell.*]

The weekly Home Practice Sheet (Handout 5.1) is given at the end of session. If MTs decide to send weekly email summaries after the group is completed, please refer to the end of Session 1 for an example of the structure of those emails. Also see Session 1 for adaptation for individual therapy.

SESSION 6

Mindful Awareness of Emotions

SESSION SUMMARY

Overview

A brief introduction is provided on emotions, including the diverse function of emotions and acceptance of emotions. In addition, there is a discussion about emotional functioning in ADHD: although core ADHD symptoms are not concerned with emotional functioning, it is increasingly recognized in the ADHD field that deficits in self-regulation of emotions play a prominent role in this condition. The R.A.I.N. exercise is introduced as a skill to help participants establish mindful awareness during times they are experiencing emotions, particularly aversive emotional states. The R.A.I.N. mnemonic stands for a series of steps to process emotions: Recognize, Accept, Investigate, and Not personalize. A sitting meditation using imagery of a recent emotionally evocative event is used as an exercise to practice this skill. Lastly, the topic of cultivating positive emotional states is introduced, including practicing a loving-kindness meditation. Participants are asked to pay attention to both positive and negative emotions in the week ahead.

Session Outline

1) Brief opening meditation exercise: Mindfulness of Thoughts (*Exercise 6.1*)
2) Review
    - Content of previous session
    - At-home practice experiences
3) Session theme: Mindful awareness of emotions
4) R.A.I.N. Introduction and Practice (*Exercise 6.2*)
5) Break

6) Walking meditation: Walking with Your Emotions (*Exercise 6.3*)
7) Cultivating positive emotions: Loving-Kindness (*Exercise 6.4*)
8) Closing
   - Discussion of home practice
   - Brief Appreciation Meditation (*Exercise 6.5*)

Home Practice

1) Formal mindfulness practice: Loving-Kindness or the R.A.I.N. exercise (15-minutes per day). Alternatively, the Walking with Your Emotions exercise.
2) Informal mindfulness practice:
   - Practicing brief informal R.A.I.N., Loving-Kindness, or Walking with Your Emotions exercises in the course of daily life.
   - Seeing how emotions come up in different situations. This can be done using the Pleasant, Unpleasant, or Neutral Events Calendar or when tracking one's ADHD patterns.

BRIEF OPENING MEDITATION EXERCISE: MINDFULNESS OF THOUGHTS

The MT starts with a brief meditation exercise that incorporates an aspect of the practice learned in the previous session on mindful awareness of thoughts. As in other sessions, this opening practice helps participants to quiet down, relax into the meeting, and become more present.

BRIEF MINDFULNESS OF THOUGHTS (5 MINUTES) (EXERCISE 6.1)

For this session's practice, we recommend a short version of the Mindfulness of Thoughts exercise.

[*Ring bell.*]

Start by finding a comfortable sitting position. Keep your back straight yet relaxed as if you are sitting in a posture of dignity. Place your hands on your lap or by your side.

Notice your breathing and allow yourself to relax in the here and now.

When your attention is relatively stable on the breath, open your awareness to thoughts you are having right now. Let the breath fall into the background and see if you can watch your thoughts float into and out of your awareness.

It may help to picture your mindful awareness as a spacious blue sky with clouds floating across it. Your awareness is like a big blue sky: vast and spacious, larger than the passing clouds. With this spacious awareness, you can watch your thoughts, feelings, and sensations as if they are clouds coming and going.

Note the content of the thoughts and the impact they may have on you while, if possible, not being drawn into thinking about them. Of course, it is easy to get lost in thinking. You may notice suddenly that you're enveloped by the cloud of thought. Whenever that occurs, shift your awareness to your breath and ground yourself in the present moment. Then, when you're ready, return to simply watching your thoughts and letting them float by.

Ask yourself, "Can I treat these thoughts for what they are: 'mental events'—no more, no less?"

[Leave about 30 seconds of silence and then ring bell.]

REVIEW

Content of Previous Session

The MT briefly discusses the formal Mindfulness of Thoughts and Walking with Your Thoughts exercises, as well as informal practices from the previous session. The previous session was focused on thoughts—whether positive or negative—and how they are associated with ADHD behaviors. Participants also discussed the role of judgmental thoughts and how they judge themselves. Participants also learned about using self-talk to guide their behavior. The MT should encourage everyone to use the handouts from the previous session to help them recall the major content and skills from the past week.

At-Home Practice Experiences

The following questions are asked to facilitate the review, starting with the informal practice (since informal practice may have been easier for participants to do during the week):

- "How many of you tracked how often you experienced judgmental thoughts since last session? For those who did, how did it go and what did you notice?"
- "Our formal meditation exercises are at 10 minutes. How did you do with that each day? Are there any 'tricks' you learned that might help others establish or maintain this routine?"
- "What were any challenges that emerged from the Mind Like a Sky or Walking with Your Thoughts exercises? What were things you liked about them?"
- "Taking a look at the big picture, have you noticed anything about how the mindfulness meditation practices and lessons behind them are beginning to impact your ADHD? In applying the lesson from last week, were you able to observe your mental states, whatever they were, without being judgmental?"
- "Were you able to do some mindful self-coaching?"

As in each session, MTs discuss the above with a balance of validation of any ongoing practice difficulties and encouragement to "stick with it."

ADAPTATION TO INDIVIDUAL THERAPY

For patients who are struggling to maintain a daily meditation schedule in the individual therapy setting, MTs may want to use a CBT technique commonly adopted in adult ADHD treatments that involves using a calendar to identify times to perform a certain behavior—in this case, meditation exercises. Any calendar that lists time increments throughout the day should work (e.g., 30-minute or 60-minute increments). Then, work with your patient to identify consistent times of the day across the week he or she is more likely meditate, and write out when that will take place in the calendar. It may help to pair up meditating with an activity the patient typically engages in already (e.g., right after a cup of coffee or tea) or make this activity contingent on meditating (i.e., self-reinforcement). Finally, collaboratively work with your patient to identify any unanticipated problems that may arise with this plan.

This adaptation can be done in a group as well, although MTs have to balance (1) providing enough support to individual participants who may be struggling to maintain a daily meditation schedule with (2) the time it takes to provide such support in a group and its impact on other participants.

SESSION THEME: MINDFUL AWARENESS OF EMOTIONS

The main theme of this session is **mindful awareness of emotions**. The session teaches how to become more aware of one's own emotions on a daily basis and how to both cope with aversive emotional states and cultivate positive emotions. The MT leads a brief psychoeducational discussion about emotions themselves. Participants are directed to Handout 6.1, which summarizes the points below.

First, emotions are described as experiences composed of three components, namely, thoughts (e.g., "What a jerk!" or "I can't stand this!"), feelings (e.g., a sense of frustration or feeling overwhelmed), and body sensations (e.g., clenched teeth or neck tension). The MT may want to draw a diagram like Figure S6.1 to illustrate the concept visually. Further, the MT should write in examples that participants provide as they discuss these different aspects of an emotional experience.

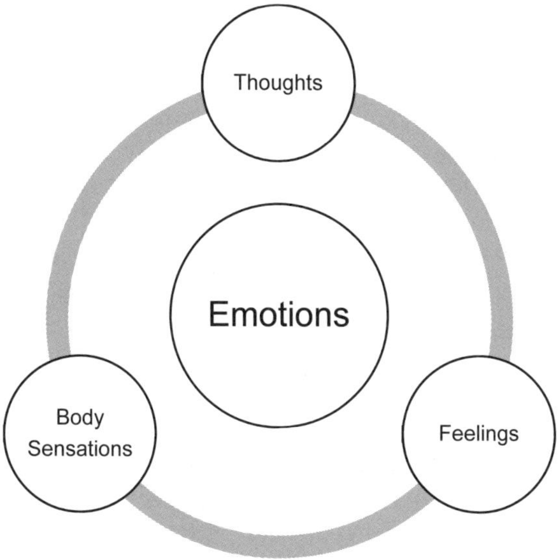

FIGURE S6.1. An illustration of different aspects of emotional experiences.

Second, both positive and negative emotions are described as universal, important, and providing useful information. Having emotions is part of being human and there's a functional purpose to them—not all negative emotions are unwanted. For example, some anxiety may motivate an individual to prepare for a particular task. When that person engages in the task, the anxiety goes down. Therefore, the anxiety can be adaptive if it contributes to completing the task at hand. At other times, that anxiety may be maladaptive if it is paralyzing and is associated with not completing the task at hand. The MT provides this example to demonstrate that negative emotions are not to be avoided, but instead they serve an important purpose. Consequently, they need to be acknowledged and accepted once they're already present, and this should all occur before deciding what else to do in response to experiencing them. Ask participants how this kind of view may differ from how they typically approach their emotional experiences.

Third, emotional states are impermanent and change over time. However, this might not be apparent to some participants, especially the more covert lingering effects once an emotion is no longer at the forefront of awareness. The MT describes how "emotions are like comets—they may have initial intensity, but they also have tails that have a residual effect." The MT can further discuss how "emotions can color our experience, even once we think they have subsided. In some cases, we may still be experiencing the residual effect of an emotion." Ask participants about how this may play out for them. One common ADHD example is mismanaging time and consequently rushing to a meeting. In the midst of rushing, a person is likely feeling stressed, tense, and fearful of being criticized. Such feelings might be most intense while rushing to the meeting, but they may linger throughout the meeting or the rest of the day. The MT then encourages participants to provide their own examples.

ADAPTATION TO INDIVIDUAL THERAPY

For patients who enjoy drawing, whether in the individual or group therapy setting, MTs might encourage patients to draw a comet and write out what this looks like in terms of their thoughts, feelings, body sensations, and actions at different points of the comet: going from the bright intense glow of the comet at the front, to the tail trailing everything else at the back. We find that sometimes taking the time to draw like this provides more time to discuss emotional experiences that allow for a richer, more contextualized narrative of how emotions are expressed for that individual.

Fourth, the MT links psychoeducation of emotions with ADHD. The MT describes how ADHD is traditionally thought of at a cognitive level (i.e., the "attention-deficit" of attention-deficit/hyperactivity disorder) and at a behavioral level (i.e., the "hyperactivity" of attention-deficit/hyperactivity disorder), but not on an emotional level. However, ADHD has an emotional component dating back to its earliest conceptualization as a disorder (see Barkley, 2010, for a review). The prominent role of poor emotion regulation in ADHD is increasingly being recognized in the research literature (e.g., Shaw, Stringaris, Nigg, & Leibenluft, 2014). For the group, the discussion should identify what emotional difficulties tend to emerge and how participants respond to them. Some symptomatic examples of poor emotion dysregulation in ADHD from Barkley (2010) include:

- Impatience
- Low frustration/intolerance
- Hot-temperedness
- Quick to anger
- Touchy or easily annoyed
- Overreactive

The MT should also check with participants to see what emotional difficulties they identify as associated with their symptoms of ADHD. For example, making careless mistakes, losing something important, or forgetting a meeting might cause frustration. As another example more typical for those with elevated hyperactive-impulsive symptoms, an adult with ADHD may feel tense or restless as they attempt to refrain from interrupting someone.

Fifth, MTs discusses how emotions in the context of ADHD might be coped with in a way that serves a functional purpose in the short term even though it's harmful to them in the long run. For example, when adults with ADHD think about a complex and/or long-term task that needs to completed, they may feel overwhelmed. One way to immediately relieve feeling overwhelmed is to do a less important, lower-priority task. This is a short-term solution (i.e., avoiding improves how the person feels) that leads to a long-term problem (i.e., the task is put off time and time again and procrastination continues).

Sixth, people with ADHD can routinely feel insecure or doubtful about themselves and their abilities after a lifetime of functional impairment associated with ADHD. Fear of rejection or shame can frequently be experienced in the context of self-doubt or, if these feelings are more covert, the person may have a tendency to be a "people pleaser," or be defensive and overreactive. With mindfulness, we want to teach participants that it is okay to approach these emotions. Mindfulness allows participants to view their own experiences with less criticism and more self-compassion, consequently enhancing ability for self-regulation. With mindfulness, there is less tendency to deny a feeling, grab onto a feeling too strongly, or emotionally overreact. Overall, mindfulness provides a choice in how one responds to a feeling. This may be best summarized by a comment commonly attributed to Viktor Frankl: "Between stimulus and response, there is a space. In that space is our power to choose our response. In our response lies our growth and freedom."

Between stimulus and response, there is a space. In that space is our power to choose our response. In our response lies our growth and freedom.

Seven, positive emotions and how they're involved with ADHD should also be acknowledged. Enthusiasm, empathy, and altruism have been noted with ADHD in popular literature, though this aspect of emotional functioning has not been thoroughly scientifically studied. Adults with ADHD may engage in impulsive enthusiasm (or become easily overexcited). Excessive excitement can lead to impulsively committing to something new while already being overcommitted. As part of a broad discussion of emotions, we encourage MTs to also ask participants if they associate positive traits or emotions with having ADHD.

Finally, MTs can discuss that a number of research studies have shown that mindfulness training is associated with experiencing lower negative emotions and more positive emotions in diverse populations (Gu, Strauss, Bond, & Cavanagh, 2015; Hölzel et al., 2011). MTs can point out that the MAPs for ADHD Program has been shown to improve emotion dysregulation in adults with ADHD (Mitchell et al., 2017).

R.A.I.N. INTRODUCTION AND PRACTICE

The MT introduces a new sitting meditation exercise: R.A.I.N. This exercise is a step-by-step guide for participants on how to recognize emotional states and how to process their emotions, and it is especially helpful for dealing with intense, aversive emotions. Each letter of the word "R.A.I.N." stands for a different step: *R* stands for Recognize, *A* stands for Accept, *I* stands for Investigate, and *N* stands for Not personalize.

The first step is **R, recognize.** Participants are invited to recognize and acknowledge the emotion while it is happening.[1] It may take some practice, but participants are encouraged to be open to notice whatever they are aware of within their inner experience, to recognize whatever emotion is present: sad, happy, excited, peaceful, tense, angry, bored, fear, embarrassment, and so on. If no obvious feeling is present, participants can notice absence of feeling, a neutral emotion, or feeling of numbness or disconnect. The MT encourages participants to name (or label) the emotions that are present: "Ah yes, there's . . . ," naming the emotion. For example, "Ah yes, there's sadness." The MT can also offer the saying, "If you name it, you can tame it."

Second is **A, accept.** After the emotion is recognized and named, this step encourages full acceptance of it. Rather than judging themselves or thinking something is wrong with them for having the emotion, participants are encouraged to allow and simply welcome the emotion. The MT reminds participants to notice and accept the emotion "as it is here, right now" without criticizing themselves for having the experience.

Third is **I, investigate.** Once participants have recognized and accepted the emotion, they can investigate it more, especially as it is felt within the body, with curiosity, openness, and interest. During the actual exercise, the MT might say something like, "What do you feel in your body? Do you feel a knotting pain in your stomach? Does your head hurt? Does your neck feel tense? . . . What kind of stories are you saying to yourself about the way you are feeling? See if you can observe them, like, 'I'm having a thought right now that this is a bad situation and it's always going to be that way.' . . . Observe what kind of emotional reactions that you are having. Do you feel angry, ashamed, and wishing you didn't feel that way?"

The final step is **N, not personalize.** *N* can also stand for *not identifying* with a particular emotion. This step may happen automatically after going through *R*, *A*, and *I*. Once participants have recognized the emotion, accepted its presence, and then

[1]While MTs tell participants that this exercise is used to process difficult emotions as they occur, the exercise in this session asks participants to perform R.A.I.N. while recalling a recent event that was emotional and aversive for them and use R.A.I.N. to process those difficult emotions retrospectively.

investigated what it feels like in the body physically, cognitively, and emotionally, they may find themselves taking the emotion less personally. They begin to see emotions as a set of sensations, thoughts, and labels. They may find themselves more as impartial observers who are less caught up in them. In this step, the MT reminds participants that emotions are transient "events" that can be watched or witnessed without having to be defined by them.

The MT should also direct participants that as they go through these steps, they should keep in mind a few different points:

- First, although this sequence is written linearly as a set of steps, often participants may go back and forth between the steps or find themselves working on some of the steps simultaneously. This is fine. The steps are guidelines and can be followed in a way that works for each person.
- Second, if it is not bearable to be with a certain emotion, participants should try to return their attention to a neutral object, like the breath or a sound. Participants should check in with themselves—if they're feeling particularly tired or unenergetic, being mindful of their emotions may be difficult.
- Third, at times when participants notice emotions and de-identify with them, they actually disappear. That's great when this occurs! However, participants are reminded that the goal here is not to get rid of emotional experiences, but to see them more clearly. The MT suggests that when we recognize and accept emotions, we often can develop some space to act more wisely.
- Finally, emotions can be difficult to work with. Intense or painful emotions especially can easily get us caught up in them. Participants are encouraged to go slowly and gently while working with emotions, and remember practicing with emotions is a lifelong task. Remind participants that memories of difficult experiences, such as dealing with death, abuse, trauma, divorce, and so on, may arise when meditating. Sometimes these memories or other experiences in meditation are too strong or painful to work with alone. We recommend that patients who notice this inform the MT, who can provide additional support or an appropriate referral. If participants notice self-harmful feelings or thoughts, it is important to address those immediately in an individualized setting, such as stepping outside of the group room—this is one reason why it is helpful to have more than one MT guiding the group.

ADAPTATION TO INDIVIDUAL THERAPY

Individual therapy is the preferred setting for those adults with ADHD who have a history of trauma, abuse, or recent or complicated grief. That is to say that for any patient who experiences very strong and overwhelming memories and emotions, individual therapy is typically the most optimal therapeutic setting. Individual attention of the therapist is often needed to help the patient process emotions without re-traumatization. The therapist may have to guide the patient out of meditation and use grounding and other trauma-informed exercises if it appears that the patient is experiencing a particularly intense or overwhelming emotion.

R.A.I.N. (EXERCISE 6.2)

In this exercise, participants are led through a meditation in which they are asked to remember a recent event during which they felt significant negative emotions, though not so strong as to be overwhelming or traumatic.

With a mindful attitude, we observe our day-to-day thoughts and feelings, like clouds floating by in the sky. Sometimes this can be difficult, especially if the clouds seem like ominous and threatening clouds from a large thunderstorm or a hurricane. The R.A.I.N. exercise can help you experience difficult emotions in a balanced way. You can say that with this practice, even if your emotions get you wet, you don't drown in them. In this practice we use the acronym R.A.I.N., which stands for: recognize, accept, investigate, and not personalize. I will guide you through each step.

Close your eyes, let your body relax, and get comfortable in your chair. Take a few deep breaths.

[*Ring bell.*]

Call to mind a past event that was stressful. Perhaps a recent difficult situation that was upsetting or frustrating. Using your mind's eye, picture where you were when this occurred, and who you were with. Recall what happened that upset you. See if you can connect with that moment by remembering details of the situation.

As you think about that event, start with the letter R and recognize whatever emotions you noticed. Use only a word or two to label what you felt: sadness, frustration, shame, hurt, anxiety, anger, embarrassment, or numbness or disconnectedness. Whatever emotion you identify is okay. Simply be curious about what you recognize.

Now, continue with the letter A, which stands for accept. See if you can radically accept what you notice. You don't have to like it or want whatever you notice, but see if you can accept or allow that this is part of your reality in this moment. Can you observe your experience without judging or critiquing yourself for having, or not having, a particular reaction? Welcome any new insights.

The next step is I, investigate. You are invited to get even closer to your experience by investigating the emotion in your body. Do you notice any sensations that are present? For example, do you feel any tension in your jaw or chest? Does your stomach feel tied up in knots? Are you clenching your teeth? Take this as an opportunity to listen to your body and see if it has anything to tell you. [*Wait about 10 seconds.*] What thoughts are present that you haven't noticed yet? What kind of narrative is going on in the background of your mind? Are there any judgments there? [*Wait about 10 seconds.*] What reactions do you have to what you're noticing? Is there any shame or frustration? [*Wait about 10 seconds.*] As you keep recognizing, accepting, and investigating your experience, remember to be kind and gentle to yourself. If this gets too difficult, it's okay to shift your attention to your breath, then return when you're ready.

Now we move on to N, not personalizing or not identifying with the difficult emotional experience. After all, emotions are a set of reactions and sensations. You are not defined by them. They are impermanent. You can simply watch your experience and learn from being with it.

[*Pause for about 30 seconds.*]

As we conclude this exercise, take a moment and see if you can offer yourself some appreciation for having the courage to be with a difficult emotion. Emotions that can feel strong or true need not have a hold on you—you can hold on to them with mindfulness.

[*Ring bell.*]

The MT invites the participants to share their experience with the above practice and uses their comments to guide the discussion. The MT encourages participants to reflect on how enhanced awareness of emotions could impact their coping with ADHD in daily life.

BREAK

This is approximately the midpoint in the session, where a 5- to 10-minute break is taken.

WALKING MEDITATION: WALKING WITH YOUR EMOTIONS

At this point we recommend a walking meditation to allow for some movement, while maintaining a focus on emotional experience. This time, in contrast to recalling a difficult memory during the first R.A.I.N. practice, the participants are asked to notice any emotion spontaneously present in the moment, even if subtle or fairly neutral.

WALKING WITH YOUR EMOTIONS (EXERCISE 6.3)

With this exercise, we are going to incorporate movement while continuing to focus on our emotional experience. Let's all stand and form a large circle. Turn to your left so that you're facing the back of the person next to you.

Let's start walking at your regular pace. [*Have the group complete one or two rotations.*]

Now stop and let your body be still and quiet. Close your eyes and feel your body standing. Feel your posture, notice your weight. Notice your energy. Check in to your body and notice if there is any tension or relaxation. Do you notice anything else in your body?

Open your eyes. Now we're going to try a slow walking meditation and focus on the sensations of moving your feet. Because we're walking in a circle, this means you have to pay attention to the person you're in front of and behind so that we don't step on each other. You may notice things like impatience bubbling up because you may want to walk differently than the person in front of you. If this happens, then it's an opportunity to practice patience and staying with your emotional experience.

Before we start walking, remember that we will be silent and focused on walking. While trying to minimize distracting things in your visual field, keep yourself aware of where you're going.

Okay, now let's begin walking slowly. Slowly lifting one leg, then the other. You may want to use your mind to label the movement as "lifting and placing, lifting and placing." You don't have to use labels to guide you, but you can if it helps you focus on your walking.

Do you observe any sensations in your feet or legs? Can you notice the sensation of movement in your body? Observe the sensation of your feet touching the ground. Note when the ball of your foot touches the floor, then when you shift your weight as you move onto the other foot. Stay connected with the sensation of walking.

[*Allow for about a minute of silent walking.*]

Now broaden your focus. While keeping your current pace, ask yourself, "What emotions are here right now?" Label these emotions with only a word or two. Rushed? Impatient? Bored? Content? Whatever you feel is okay.

If you notice or recognize any emotion that you don't want to experience, ask yourself if you can let it stay. Can you radically accept that it is here? As you walk, see if you can carry the emotion with you and let it be part of your journey.

Can you get closer to the emotion and investigate it closer? Where do you feel it in your body? Are there any thoughts that accompany the emotion?

See if you can let go of personalizing the experience. Instead, see it as something that's not permanent, but passing. Can you see it as a set of sensations that don't define you, that are not you?

[*Allow for about a minute of silent walking.*]

Now stop walking and allow your eyes to close. How are you feeling? Is there something new you noticed in this practice? Whatever your experience is—positive, negative, or neutral—it is okay. See if you can accept the present experience however it is.

Take a moment to congratulate yourself for practicing noticing your emotions. Take a deep breath, and when you feel ready, go ahead and open your eyes.

Next, the MT asks participants about their experiences with the exercise. Some may notice that their experience was similar to the sitting R.A.I.N. exercise, while others may notice differences. The MT should suggest that mindful walking may be a more appropriate fit than the sitting R.A.I.N. exercise at times when there is a lot of restlessness. The MT can also encourage participants to challenge themselves and practice the R.A.I.N. exercise while sitting.

CULTIVATING POSITIVE EMOTIONS: LOVING-KINDNESS

Up until this point in the session, the discussion has primarily focused around how to cope with aversive emotional states. However, MTs will also want to emphasize that we're not just trying to be with what's aversive, but also trying to build upon positive emotional experiences in daily life as well. We accomplish this by teaching participants about self-compassion and practicing a loving-kindness exercise to build up positive emotional experiences. Mindfulness practices, especially loving-kindness exercises, are proposed to help participants reappraise stressful events so that they are less overwhelming. When that occurs, participants are better at decentering (i.e., the process of de-identification from thoughts, feelings, and sensations) from stressful events. In turn, this elicits greater mindfulness (e.g., letting go of judgment) and enhances attentional functioning, resulting in greater likelihood of cultivating greater positive emotional experiences (see Garland et al., 2010, for more discussion on upward spirals of emotional experiences).

LOVING-KINDNESS (EXERCISE 6.4)[2]

This is a traditional loving-kindness exercise is also known as "metta meditation" or directing well-wishes toward the self and toward other people.

Settle into a comfortable sitting position. Take a couple of deep breaths and relax your body.

[*Ring bell.*]

In this practice, you are invited to cultivate positive emotions such as friendliness, love, kindness, and compassion for yourself and others. This isn't always easy, and it can feel a bit unnatural at first. Simply be open to what happens to you during this practice, noticing your experience from moment to moment.

Bring to your mind a person in your life who easily evokes feelings of love and warmth: maybe a child, your significant other, or even a pet. Imagine them standing in front of you.

Notice how you feel as you bring them to mind. There may be a feeling of happiness or warmth in your body, a smile on your face, or a sense of an open heart. This feeling is loving-kindness—a feeling of caring and friendliness.

As you imagine your loved one, see if you can silently wish him or her happiness and well-being. You can use words such as "May you be happy, may you be safe, may you be healthy and live with ease." Or come up with your own phrases reflecting love and kindness.

Gently repeat the wishes of well-being several times. As you do, continue to notice how your body feels.

If at any point you find that your attention has wandered off, gently bring it back and begin again.

Now see if you can extend the wishes of loving-kindness to yourself. You may repeat words like "May I be happy, may I be safe, may I be healthy and live with ease. May I accept myself as I am." Or use your own words.

Notice how it feels to extend caring wishes to yourself. If you notice that you're not feeling anything, or that you're feeling something else other than loving-kindness, just bring curiosity to that. Notice what's arising in your thoughts and in your body. You can learn from this experience, no matter what it's like.

Traditionally, loving-kindness is extended in stages, starting with oneself and extending to those we love, those we feel neutral about, those we consider our enemies, and then all beings.

See if you can send out loving-kindness to other people in your life. Imagine opening your heart and extending loving-kindness in all directions: to people you care about, people whom you feel neutral about or don't know, and people who are suffering. Touch them with thoughts such as "May we all be happy; may we all be safe, healthy, and live with ease; may we all be compassionate and gentle with ourselves and others; may we all experience joy and well-being."

See if you can extend loving-kindness to people you find difficult or who have harmed you in some way. See what comes up for you and observe whether you're ready to send such wishes.

---

[2]Adapted and reprinted with permission from *The Mindfulness Prescription for Adult ADHD* (Zylowska, 2012).

Take a moment to congratulate yourself for practicing loving-kindness. Take a deep breath, and when you feel ready, go ahead and open your eyes.

[*Ring bell.*]

During this discussion, the MT brings up the concept of cultivating different positive emotions, much like we did in this exercise. The analogy of "watering our seeds" is introduced (adapted from Hanh, 2001)—Do participants water the seeds of anger, criticism, blame, or distraction? Or, do they water seeds of tolerance, love, and compassion for self and others? When participants practice loving-kindness exercises, they nurture the latter. The MT also introduces a brief gesture of self-compassion—placing your hand over your heart—as an alternative way to connect with the intention of love, kindness, and compassion for yourself in daily life, and especially in the midst of a difficulty. The MT can also add discussion of other positive emotional states, such as gratitude, joy, accomplishment, or contentment (including a sense of accomplishment after finishing a task, for example). The MT can suggest "catching yourself doing well," taking in the feeling of willingness to do something or a feeling of mastery. Other topics, such as humor and forgiveness, can be brought in or elicited from the group.

CLOSING

Discussion of Home Practice

The MT should make sure to take sufficient time to review the plan for exercises to complete at home. This time is used to address questions, clarify any points of confusion, and "fill in the blanks" for any participants who may have experienced mind wandering during parts of the session or those who feel unsure about what is being asked of them in the week ahead. These are the basic points to convey (also summarized in Handout 6.2).

The formal practice is either the Loving-Kindness or the R.A.I.N. exercise for 15 minutes per day. Alternatively, participants can also use the Walking with Your Emotions exercise.

There are two informal practices for this week:

1. To process any difficult emotional experiences that may come up during your daily life, practice brief informal versions of R.A.I.N., Loving-Kindness, or Walking with Your Emotions exercises. See Handout 6.3 for a summary of R.A.I.N.
2. See how your emotions come up in different situations. Consider using the Pleasant, Unpleasant, or Neutral Events Calendar (Handout 6.4) or the previous Handout 2.3 to track your reactions.

BRIEF APPRECIATION MEDITATION (EXERCISE 6.5)

At the close of this session, introduce a short meditation lasting about 2 minutes that includes a moment to stop and reflect on the session just completed and appreciation for participants, including themselves. Invite participants to offer appreciation, compassion, or loving-kindness to themselves for making the time to practice mindfulness and self-care, and offer appreciation to others for their presence in the class. The short closing meditation allows participants to experience positive emotions and gratefulness. Here's how the exercise might be narrated:

> We close with a short appreciation practice. Sit in a relaxed yet upright posture and either close your eyes or keep them resting in one spot.
>
> [*Ring bell.*]
>
> Take a moment to appreciate everyone's presence today. People attending the group are here to care for themselves or to better their situations. The reasons may differ, but everyone is here to grow and improve their lives. Also, bring a sense of appreciation or compassion to yourself, for being here and taking the time for learning about yourself and mindfulness. See if you can connect with a sense of appreciation and gratitude in your body as you offer it to others and yourself.
>
> [*Ring bell.*]

Depending on factors like the amount of time left in the session, for a slightly longer version of this exercise that incorporates components of loving-kindness mindfulness meditation, you may want to incorporate the following into the exercise above:

> In your mind, say the following to others: "May you be happy, may you be safe, may you be healthy and live with ease." [*Repeat this line two or three more times.*]
>
> Avoid forcing a sense of appreciation. Instead, simply ask yourself if it's there already. If it's not there, just setting the intention to appreciate the presence of others is important.
>
> Now, take a moment and offer yourself loving-kindness for making the time to practice mindfulness and take care of yourself, which will then help you take care of others and situations once you walk out of this room.
>
> In your mind, say the following to yourself: "May I be happy, may I be safe, may I be healthy and live with ease." [*Repeat this line two or three more times.*]
>
> Take this feeling of appreciation with you, but before you mentally leave the room, take this moment to sit and allow yourself to experience the positive emotion and a sense of gratefulness.
>
> Let it spread in your body and move outward with you as you move on to the next part of your day.
>
> [*Ring bell.*]

The weekly Home Practice Sheet (Handout 6.2) is given at the end of session. If MTs decide to send weekly email summaries after the group is completed, please refer to the end of Session 1 for an example of the structure of those emails. Also see Session 1 for adaptation for individual therapy.

SESSION 7

Mindful Awareness of Presence and Interactions

SESSION SUMMARY

Overview

Mindful awareness of interactions with others is addressed in this session. Difficulties in social awareness and social interactions are frequently found in ADHD—including not listening, interrupting, talking too much, blurting out answers, or being distracted in a conversation—and this session teaches mindful listening and mindful speech. As prelude to the practice, and a way to bring together what has been learned so far, an exercise called Mindful Presence (also known as Open Awareness or Choiceless Awareness) is introduced. Parallels are drawn to different attentional aspects (e.g., alerting, orienting, conflict attention, as well as single-focus and receptive attention). In the second part of the session, the participants partner up to practice an exercise in which one person is the sole speaker while the other one is the sole listener. The speaker is asked to reflect on a topic and "speak from the heart" while the listener is to simply listen and bring awareness to his or her automatic responses, such as an urge to interrupt or comment. Outside of the session, participants are asked to practice similar mindful speaking and listening with a friend or a spouse.

Session Outline

1) Brief opening meditation exercise: R.A.I.N. (*Exercise 7.1*)
2) Review
   - Content of previous session
   - At-home practice experiences
3) Session theme: Mindful awareness of presence and interactions

4) Mindful Presence Introduction and Practice (*Exercise 7.2*)
5) Discussion of different facets of single-focus attention versus receptive attention
6) Break
7) Short Walking Meditation (*Exercise 7.3*)
8) Mindful awareness of interactions
9) Mindful Listening and Speaking (*Exercise 7.4*)
10) Closing
    - Discussion of home practice
    - Brief Appreciation Meditation (*Exercise 7.5*)

Home Practice

1) Formal mindfulness practice: Daily 15-minute sitting meditation: Mindful Presence
2) Informal mindfulness practice:
    - Mindful speaking and listening with a spouse or a friend
    - Listening mindfully during regular conversation in daily life
    - Noticing with curiosity interactions with other people

BRIEF OPENING MEDITATION EXERCISE: R.A.I.N.

The MT opens class with an abbreviated R.A.I.N. meditation.

R.A.I.N. PRACTICE (5 MINUTES) (EXERCISE 7.1)

[*Ring bell.*]

Find your posture, back against the chair, arms in a comfortable position. Close your eyes or keep them resting in one spot.

Take a few deep breaths to settle into the present moment.

Using the acronym R.A.I.N.—recognize, accept, investigate, and not personalize—we now practice checking into with ourselves, noticing any feelings, even subtle ones that may be present right now.

First, bring awareness to your mind and body and recognize what feelings may be present. There may be feelings that are pleasant, unpleasant, or fairly neutral. Perhaps a sense of rushing and worry or perhaps a feeling of relaxation and ease. There may be feelings of excitement, confidence, or boredom or doubt. You may also notice a rather neutral emotional state.

Whatever you notice, see if you can accept or allow your experience fully. Even if you don't like what you are noticing, see if you can practice accepting what is already here, in the moment.

Spend some time investigating your feelings a bit more, noticing any body sensations or thoughts that may be associated with the feeling. If the feelings are subtle or neutral, notice what your body is like during this state.

[*Pause for about 1–2 minutes.*]

Finally, remember that our feelings are just feelings. They are reactions and inner experiences that we can watch and not personalize. We don't have to be driven by our feelings—we can witness them, hold them in awareness, and let them pass.

[*Leave about 30 seconds of silence and then ring bell.*]

REVIEW

Content of Previous Session

The MT reviews the previous session's focus on observing and accepting emotions via the practice of R.A.I.N., as well as fostering self-compassion and positive emotional experiences. Loving-kindness practice and the intention of self-compassion are briefly reviewed as a way to buffer negative emotional experiences.

At-Home Practice Experiences

The following questions are asked to facilitate the homework review:

- "Were you mindful of emotions in your practice or in daily life?"
- "Were you able to practice the loving-kindness meditation during the week?"
- "What difficulties have you noticed with your practice this week?"
- "Any insights or successes with the practice?"

The MT encourages participants to review and share from their at-home practice tracking sheets.

SESSION THEME: MINDFUL AWARENESS OF PRESENCE AND INTERACTIONS

Mindful presence toward one's inner experience and when being with others are discussed as keys to effective communication. This topic is tied to common difficulties in social interactions and social awareness found in ADHD. First we explore by bringing together the elements of mindful practice learned so far and then we apply those in an exercise called Mindful Presence (also known as Open Awareness or Choiceless Awareness). Whereas the formal mindfulness meditation exercises thus far have been more directed and focused, this is an open monitoring exercise. Such progression from focused to open monitoring exercises is typically used in mindfulness-based interventions (Davidson & Kaszniak, 2015). It is thought that monitoring skills developed through focused exercises help people engage in open awareness practice without easily succumbing to being lost in thought or rumination. The open awareness practice invites participants to be aware and open to whatever arises in the present moment, be it breath, sound, body sensations, thoughts, or feelings. This is initially practiced in a silent sitting meditation and later related to relational mindfulness or mindfulness in interactions with others. Since this formal practice is 15 minutes—longer than previous formal practices—only a brief introduction of the session theme is used here. Also, at this point the participants have familiarity with the basic elements of formal meditation and, thus, application of these elements via experiential learning is emphasized here.

MINDFUL PRESENCE INTRODUCTION AND PRACTICE

A brief segue into the Mindful Presence exercise might be something like, "We're going to practice an exercise in which you are invited to be aware and open to whatever arises in the present moment. We'll discuss this more after the practice, so for now let's go ahead and dive in."

MINDFUL PRESENCE (EXERCISE 7.2)[1]

The ability to be fully present to ourselves and to another person requires a flexible and receptive attention. In this practice, called open or choiceless awareness, we practice noticing whatever arises from moment to moment and noticing the changing flow of experience within us and outside of us.

Begin by sitting comfortably in an upright position. Briefly scan your body and relax any areas of tension. Close your eyes.

[*Ring bell.*]

Gently bring the attention to your breath. Notice the movement of the breath in its natural state. Remember the breath is always there, in the present. You can always return to it if you get lost in feeling or thinking.

[*Pause.*]

Now, set the intention to be aware, welcoming, or receptive to whatever arises in each moment. Allow things to come and go at their own speed as you rest in the present moment.

If a sound becomes obvious, open your attention to allow awareness of that sound alongside your breathing. If the sound pulls your attention away from the breath, place your full attention on the sound and allow your breathing to fall into the background. You may choose to name or label the experience several times before the experience passes. For example, noting to yourself "hearing, hearing, hearing, hearing" for the duration of the sound. Listen to the sound until it no longer holds your attention, then return to the breath.

If a body sensation arises, open your attention to it and hold both the sensation and your breathing together in awareness. If the sensation strongly pulls your attention away from the breath, turn your full attention to it and allow your breath to fall into the background.

Explore the physical sensation. Is it itching? Burning? Vibrations? Pressure? Contraction or expansion? Changing? Staying the same? When the sensation no longer holds your attention, again simply return to your breathing or allow something else to arise in its place.

If an emotion becomes obvious, as with any other sensation, open your attention to it alongside your breathing. If the emotion strongly pulls your attention, turn your full attention to it and allow your breath to fall into the background. If you wish, you can use the R.A.I.N. practice to observe the emotion. Recognizing and accepting what is happening, and investigating and not personalizing or identifying with it. Label the emotion and check in to your body. Perhaps

[1]Partially adapted and reprinted with permission from *The Mindfulness Prescription for Adult ADHD* (Zylowska, 2012).

there is fluttering or uneasiness in the belly. Perhaps there is a feeling of impatience. Notice the emotion with curiosity. When the emotion is no longer strong, bring your attention back to your breath or whatever else is obvious in the present moment.

If a thought or image comes to your awareness, acknowledge its presence as you continue breathing. Many times thoughts remain in the background and you can be aware of them coming and going like clouds in a sky. If you get lost in thinking, once you notice the lapse in awareness, gently return to the breath. However, if a thought is obsessive and keeps coming back, bring your full attention to it and allow your breath to fade into the background. Label the type of thought, such as worry, planning, or judgment. Check in to the body and see if there are any emotions or body sensations as well. When ready, return to the breath.

You may also notice other things, maybe a general state of energy, your alertness level, an attitude or mood.

Allow each experience until it shifts to the next one. You don't have to hold on to anything or make anything happen. Simply relax and open, allowing what is unfolding. Practice connecting with the experience and letting it go on its own accord.

Continue this in silence with your awareness open and receptive.

[*Pause for about 1 minute.*]

As we end, give yourself appreciation for sitting through this practice of awareness. Extend loving kindness to yourself and wish yourself well. May I be happy, may I be safe, may I be healthy and live with ease. May I be present and compassionate to myself and others.

[*Pause for about 1 minute.*]

Extend these wishes to all people. May we all be happy, may we all be safe, may we all be healthy and live with ease. May we all experience true listening and compassion in each other.

[*Ring bell.*]

The MT invites participants to share their experience with open awareness practice.

DISCUSSION OF DIFFERENT FACETS OF ATTENTION AND SINGLE-FOCUS VERSUS RECEPTION ATTENTION

As part of the discussion, the MT reviews different facets of attention discussed in past sessions (i.e., alerting, orienting, conflict), and the difference between single-focus exercises versus receptive exercises. The following points are incorporated:

- Alerting has to do with *readying or gearing up attention* to respond to experiences. It also involves maintaining good alertness over time. Vigilance and alertness/arousal are related to this facet. The difference in the brightness or readiness of your attention is a difference in alerting—think about when you are tired versus when you are well rested.
- Orienting has to do with *movement of attention* toward a sensory stimulus or shifting attention from one thing to another. As an example, reading and moving your attention from one side of the page to the other is engaging this facet.
- Conflict has to do with choosing and controlling responses, and it is involved in *paying attention despite distractions.*

- We understand from research studies that alerting and conflict are typically more impaired in ADHD than orienting is.
- These facets of attention are most readily experienced with a single-focus attention such as Mindfulness of Breathing.
- Open awareness or receptive attention has to do with openness to the flow of experiences in the present moment. In the single-focus exercises we started with, we focus on something in particular, like the breath or a sound, and we keep returning to that anchor of attention. In open awareness or receptive attention you allow whatever arises to be in your awareness, thus it is also called "choiceless awareness."
- Research supports that both focused and open awareness exercises cultivate multiple aspects of attention to improve overall psychological well-being (Wolkin, 2015).

Since the open awareness practice is the longest meditation in the MAPs for ADHD Program training and it can generate longer discussion, the MT can decide at this point to take a break and practice the walking meditation afterward. For larger groups, the Mindful Listening and Speaking exercise will also take longer, and the MT may choose to move to that right after the break.

BREAK

This is approximately the midpoint in the session, where a 5- to 10-minute break is taken.

SHORT WALKING MEDITATION

OPTIONAL SHORT WALKING MEDITATION (EXERCISE 7.3)

Let's form a big circle.

Close your eyes and let your body be still and quiet. Keep your feet together and feel your body standing.

Feel your posture, notice your weight, and if there is any tension or pain or maybe good feelings, too.

Now open your eyes and rest them just a short distance in front of you. Avoid looking around, as it can be distracting; however, keep yourself aware of where you are going.

We're going to walk slowly in a circle and focus on the sensations of moving your feet. You may also choose to focus on the sensations at the very bottom of your feet as you place them on the ground.

Ready? Let's begin. Slowly lift one of your legs and begin to walk. In your mind, you can label the movement as "lifting and placing" "lifting and placing" *or* simply observe the movement without labeling.

As you walk, you can also notice the sensations of your feet touching the ground; noting the placement of the ball of the foot and the shift in weight and balance as you walk.

If you like, synchronize your breathing with your footsteps. For example, as you step with one foot, inhale; as you step with the other foot, exhale.

If your mind wanders, gently bring your attention back to the sensations at the soles of your feet.

[*Pause.*]

Where is your attention right now? If you need to, bring it back to lifting and placing your feet or to the bottom of your feet.

Now, stop and close your eyes. Feel your whole body and notice how you feel inside. Is there is a sense of impatience or wanting to rush? Or perhaps you notice a sense of relaxation. Open your awareness to whatever is present within you or outside of you. Simply notice whatever your experience is with openness, kindness, and curiosity.

[*Pause and then ring bell.*]

MINDFUL AWARENESS OF INTERACTIONS

The MT reviews ADHD-related cognitive or behavioral symptoms, pointing out in a nonjudgmental way the behaviors that can interfere with effective or satisfying communication (see Handout 7.1). Examples include interrupting, not listening, talking too much, or blurting things out.

The MT discusses how ADHD-influenced communication behaviors can lead to others' frustration and, at the same time, leave the person with ADHD feeling misunderstood, criticized, or isolated. The MT brings up how communication difficulties are often described in families and romantic relationships affected with ADHD. Acknowledgment of the neural basis of ADHD-associated behaviors, mindful awareness, compassion, and accountability are discussed as necessary components of working through such difficulties. Ask participants if they tend to be to-the point in conversations or if they tend to talk a lot. You might want to draw out a typical communication challenge in ADHD similar to Figure S7.1. In Figure S7.1, we use the example of coworkers talking about if they're going to a meeting. Conversation A is efficient and linear, whereas Conversation B is much more tangential. Drawing an interaction out in this way may help participants process how interaction with someone with ADHD typically proceeds. We recommend using group member comments to guide your illustration. The main point is to identify how ADHD may lead to conversations that are off topic, given the executive functions deficits and verbal impulsivity found in the disorder.

MINDFUL LISTENING AND SPEAKING

The Mindfulness of Listening and Speaking practice is offered next as a way to practice awareness in interactions.

MINDFUL LISTENING AND SPEAKING (EXERCISE 7.4)

In this exercise, each participant will sit facing another participant and listen to them talk for 5 minutes about a subject. We recommend that the MT suggests a topic such

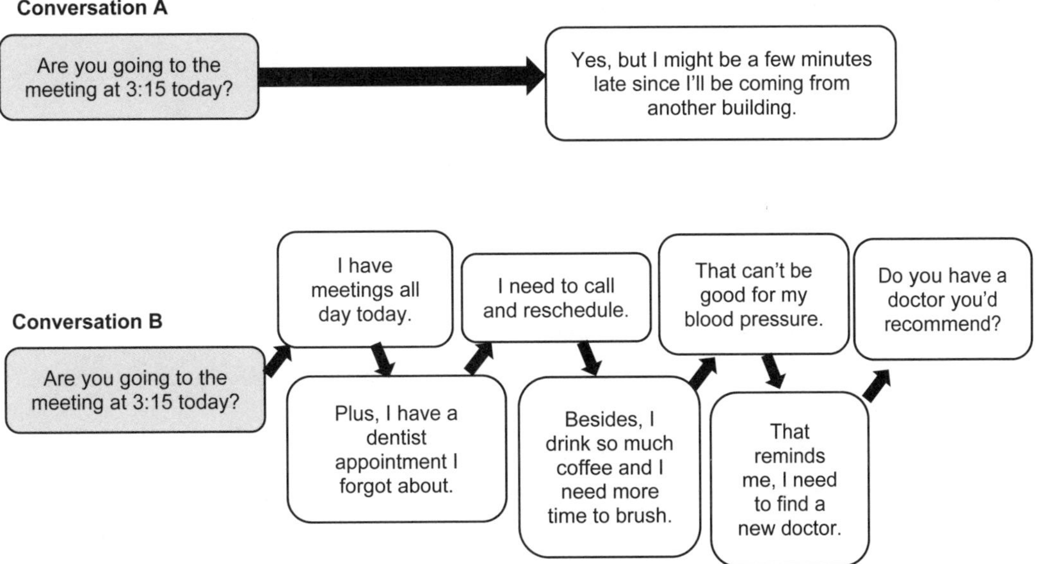

FIGURE S7.1. The flow of conversations: succinct (Conversation A) and tangential (Conversation B).

as (1) discuss how you feel about having ADHD or (2) discuss your main frustrations when communicating with others. Next the MT sets guidelines for the interaction:

- *The listeners* will practice openness and deep listening. This means being nonjudgmental and giving the speakers their full attention, practicing not interrupting, and noticing if they feel distracted, bored, critical, or eager to jump in.
- *The speakers* will practice mindful speaking with the intention to "speak from the heart." Such speaking includes awareness of one's body and emotions, and practicing not getting distracted from the core topic. After 5 minutes the MT will ring the bell and the pair will switch roles.
- After each participant has played each role once, they will share with each other and the group about the full experience.
- Participants will begin the practice breathing, relaxing their body, and coming back to the intention to communicate mindfully.

After the above exercise is done in dyads, the MT invites the participants to share with the whole group their observations. The MT models curiosity and nonjudgment and can use these prompts to facilitate the reflection for the listening part of the exercise:

- "How was it being a sole listener?"
- "Did you have any urges to interrupt?"

- "When listening, were you able to stay focused throughout the whole 5 minutes?"
- "Did you miss any part of the conversation?"
- "Did you use any strategies to help you stay focused and fully engaged?"
- "How did you feel during this part of the practice? Did you notice being relaxed or tense? Engaged or distracted?"

For the speaking part of the exercise, the following prompts can be used:

- "How was it being the sole speaker?"
- "Did you notice how easy or hard it was to express yourself during this exercise?"
- "How did you feel during this part of the practice?"
- "Did you notice anything about your communication style?"

Refer participants to Handout 7.2 for directions on how to practice this skill as a home practice.

ADAPTATION TO INDIVIDUAL THERAPY

The topic of mindful communication in ADHD can be expanded beyond the content provided in the group setting. The individual therapist can bring Marshall Rosenberg's nonviolent or compassionate communication model (Rosenberg, 1999) to the sessions and practice using this with the patient. The model emphasizes nonjudgmental stating of facts and using "I" statements with a focus on feelings, needs, and specific requests. Modeling and rehearsing in session on how to address a current conflict in a relationship can be also very helpful to patients with ADHD who have a maladaptive communication style (e.g., blaming others) or have trouble connecting with and expressing their own feelings and needs.

Another topic to check into is sensitivity to rejection and criticism (or related, a "people pleasing" habit that often forms to avoid experiencing rejection or criticism). This sensitivity has been noted in the ADHD field as relevant to people with ADHD, and can contribute to communication difficulties. The MT can also explore communication topics (e.g., not listening) in the context of a patient's romantic relationship or in parent–child relationships affected by ADHD. See Handout 8.5 for selected books by Melissa Orlov, Gina Pera, and Gabor Mate.

CLOSING

Discussion of Home Practice

The MT should make sure to take sufficient time to review the plan for exercises to complete at home. This time is used to address questions, clarify any points of confusion, and "fill in the blanks" for any participants who may have experienced mind wandering during parts of the session or those who feel unsure about what is being asked of them in the week ahead. These are the basic points to convey (also summarized in Handout 7.3).

The formal practice is the 15-minute Mindful Presence exercise daily.
There are three informal practices for this week.

1. Ask a friend, family member, or spouse to do a mindfulness exercise with you. Either (1) review Handout 7.1 with them and get their feedback, or (2) find one time to practice mindful listening and speaking with that person.
2. Participants are also encouraged to listen mindfully when engaged in regular conversations with others in the course of the week.
3. We also ask participants to pay attention to their interactions and consider using optional Handout 2.3 to build on "putting things together" that were also learned in previous sessions.

BRIEF APPRECIATION MEDITATION (EXERCISE 7.5)

At the close of this session, introduce a short meditation lasting about 2 minutes that includes a moment to stop and reflect on the session just completed and appreciation for participants, including themselves. Invite participants to offer appreciation or loving-kindness to themselves for making the time to practice mindfulness and self-care, and offer appreciation to others for their presence in the class. The short closing meditation allows participants to experience positive emotions and gratefulness. Here's how the exercise might be narrated:

> We close with a short appreciation practice. Sit in a relaxed yet upright posture and either close your eyes or keep them resting in one spot.
>
> [*Ring bell.*]
>
> Take a moment to appreciate everyone's presence today. People attending the group are here to care for themselves or to better their situations. The reasons may differ, but everyone is here to grow and improve their lives. Also, bring a sense of appreciation to yourself, for being here and taking the time for learning about yourself and mindfulness. See if you can connect with a sense of appreciation and gratitude in your body as you offer it to others and yourself.
>
> [*Ring bell.*]

Depending on factors like amount of time left in the session, for a slightly longer version of this exercise that incorporates components of loving-kindness mindfulness meditation, you may want to incorporate the following into the exercise above.

> In your mind, say the following to others: "May you be happy, may you be safe, may you be healthy and live with ease." *[Repeat this line two or three more times.]*
>
> Avoid forcing a sense of appreciation. Instead, simply ask yourself if it's there already. If it's not there, just setting the intention to appreciate the presence of others is important.
>
> Now, take a moment and offer yourself loving-kindness for making the time to practice mindfulness and take care of yourself, which will then help you take care of others and situations once you walk out of this room.
>
> In your mind, say the following to yourself: "May I be happy, may I be safe, may I be healthy and live with ease." [*Repeat this line two or three more times.*]

Take this feeling of appreciation with you, but before you mentally leave the room, take this moment to sit and allow yourself to experience the positive emotion and a sense of gratefulness.

Let it spread in your body and move outward with you as you move on to the next part of your day.

[*Ring bell.*]

The weekly Home Practice Sheet (Handout 7.3) is given at the end of session. If MTs decide to send weekly email summaries after the group is completed, please refer to the end of Session 1 for an example of the structure of those emails. Also see Session 1 for adaptation for individual therapy.

SESSION 8

Mindful Awareness as a Life Journey

SESSION SUMMARY

Overview

The theme of this session is to review the MAPs for ADHD training and emphasize ways to integrate mindful awareness as a part of daily life with ADHD. The mindful awareness concepts and practices taught in the MAPs for ADHD Program are reviewed, and resources for ongoing mindful awareness practice are provided. In the first part of the session, participants sit in a 20-minute mindful presence mediation, which is followed by a 10-minute mindful walking practice. This is done to give participants experience with longer mindfulness practice. In the second part of the session, participants are invited to comment on what they learned in the process of the class. Such reflection can be done during a "speaking council" exercise in which everyone has a chance to share their experience. Learning mindfulness is framed as a lifelong process of checking in with one's attention, renewing the intention to return to the present moment, and applying the acceptance–change dialectic each day. Environmental modifications derived from ADHD coaching and CBT approaches are reviewed to help participants remember being mindful or practice loving-kindness. Additional resources about ADHD and/or mindfulness are provided, such as books, websites, and other mindfulness-based classes.

Session Outline

1) Brief opening meditation exercise: S.T.O.P. (*Exercise 8.1*)
2) Review
    - Content of previous session
    - At-home practice experiences

3) Session theme: Mindful awareness as a life journey
4) Mindful Presence (*Exercise 8.2*) and Walking Meditation (*Exercise 8.3*)
5) Break
6) Review of covered mindfulness principles
7) Beyond MAPs: ADHD and mindfulness resources
8) Closing Ceremony (*Exercise 8.4*)

BRIEF OPENING MEDITATION EXERCISE: S.T.O.P.

The MT welcomes participants and begins with a short breathing meditation that reviews the concept of mindful presence from the previous session. The MT leads participants through a short S.T.O.P. meditation, which was first introduced in Session 3, and starts with the breath as an anchor and then expands awareness to observe all experiences that arise, including thoughts, feelings, sound, and body sensations. As an alternative to this opening exercise, MTs may also consider the Breathing Space exercise commonly covered in MBCT (see Segal et al., 2002, p. 174, for an example of a narration).

BRIEF S.T.O.P. PRACTICE (5 MINUTES) (EXERCISE 8.1)

Sit comfortably and close your eyes.

[*Ring bell.*]

Today we will use the S.T.O.P. practice to bring mindful presence into moments of our lives.

In this practice, the letter *S* reminds us to stop or pause. Let go of busy thinking or doing.

The letter *T* reminds us to take a few deeper breaths. Anchor your attention on the sensations of the breath coming in and going out.

Next, the letter *O* reminds us to observe in the present moment. See if you can open your awareness to notice anything else that is here: any sounds, body sensations, thoughts, feelings, needs. Observe the stream of experiences coming and going, noticing the shifts in your awareness and coming back to the breath as the anchor if you find yourself distracted or caught in thinking.

[*Pause.*]

As we end the meditation, the letter *P* reminds us, we can proceed into the next moment now with more awareness.

[*Leave about 30 seconds of silence and then ring bell.*]

REVIEW

Content of Previous Session

The MT reviews the previous session's focus on increasing awareness of interactions, including the Mindful Listening and Speaking exercise. The Mindful Presence exercise is also reviewed.

At-Home Practice Experiences

The MT asks participants to use their tracking sheets to reflect on the past week's practice. The following questions are asked to facilitate the homework review:

- "How was your practice this week?"
- "Did you practice mindful presence?"
- "How about mindful speaking and listening?"

SESSION THEME: MINDFUL AWARENESS AS A LIFE JOURNEY

In moving forward, the MT frames mindfulness as a life journey or lifelong practice of:

1. Checking in with one's attention and returning to the present moment throughout the day.
2. Applying the acceptance–change dialectic in each day.
3. Renewing the intention to practice mindfulness if the practice goes by the wayside for some time.

The MT also highlights additional points. First, the MT frames mindfulness practice as training the skill of regularly pausing and observing what's going on in the present moment, either inside or outside of us. This skill requires repetition in the same way physical training and training for any other skills do. For example, it takes 50 hours to learn the harmonica and 1,200 hours to learn play the violin (Strayhorn, 2002).

Second, the MT asks participants to challenge themselves and lean with curiosity and kindness into negative experiences to transform them. For example, the MT might say:

> "Check in with yourself when you want to procrastinate, feel bored, get angry, cannot remember something, etc. Be present in the moment—get in closer and check in about how you feel. Ask yourself about what emotion, body sensations, thoughts, etc. are present. Ask yourself 'What are the barriers?' and 'What intention would I like to set?' "

Third, the MT asks participants to remember to practice self-acceptance and compassion, as well as mindful self-coaching to transform ADHD-related challenges and mitigate shame and self-doubt that often accompany ADHD. The MT also encourages participants to intentionally connect and take in positive emotions such as appreciation of self and others, gratitude, humor, and joy.

Fourth, the MT acknowledges that being consistent with practicing awareness and loving-kindness in daily life is often difficult. The practice itself is typically not as hard as remembering and staying motivated to keep doing it. Therefore, reminders and other ways to keep motivated are very important. The MT makes several suggestions of strategies to make mindfulness part of one's life. The suggestions are in Handout 8.1

and Handout 8.2, both of which the MT reviews with the group. The participants are encouraged to circle the suggestions that they would like to incorporate into their life after the class is finished.

MINDFUL PRESENCE AND WALKING MEDITATION

Experiencing Longer Mindfulness Practices

In the first part of the session, the MT leads a sitting mindful presence meditation (20 minutes). This is followed by a mindful walking practice (10 minutes). The practices incorporate all key elements learned in the previous sessions. Overall, the silent practice is about 30 minutes, giving participants the longest experience with meditation practice so far in the MAPs for ADHD course.

MINDFUL PRESENCE (EXERCISE 8.2)[1]

Begin by sitting comfortably in an upright position. Briefly scan your body and relax any areas of tension. Close your eyes.

[*Ring bell.*]

Gently bring attention to your breath. Notice the movement of the breath in its natural state. Remember the breath is always there, in the present. You can always return to it if you get lost in feeling or thinking.

[*Pause.*]

Now, set the intention to be aware and receptive to whatever arises in each moment . . . in a choiceless and welcoming way.

If a sound becomes obvious, open your attention to allow awareness of that sound alongside your breathing. If the sound pulls your attention away from the breath, place your full attention on the sound and allow your breathing to fall into the background. As your concentration strengthens, mindfulness gets brighter. You might find that you note or label several times before the event or experience passes. For example, you might note "hearing, hearing, hearing, hearing" for the duration of the experience. Allow things to move at their own speed. Events come and go and you rest in the present moment. Listen to the sound until it no longer holds your attention, then return to the breath.

If a body sensation arises, open your attention to it and hold both the sensation and your breathing together in awareness. If the sensation strongly pulls your attention away from the breath, turn your full attention to it and allow your breath to fall into the background. Explore the physical sensation. Is it itching? Burning? Vibrations? Pressure? Contraction or expansion? Changing? Staying the same? When the sensation no longer holds your attention, again simply return to your breathing—the anchor of awareness. Feeling the experience deeply for as long as it's here, and letting it go as something else takes its place.

If an emotion becomes obvious, as with any other sensation, open your attention to it alongside your breathing. If the emotion strongly pulls your attention, turn your full attention to it and allow your breath to fall into the background. If you wish, you can use the R.A.I.N. practice to observe the emotion. Recognizing and accepting what is happening, and investigating

[1]Partially adapted and reprinted with permission from *The Mindfulness Prescription for Adult ADHD* (Zylowska, 2012).

and not personalizing or not identifying with it. Label the emotion and check in to your body. Perhaps there is fluttering or uneasiness in the belly. Perhaps there is a feeling of impatience. Notice the emotion with curiosity. When the emotion is no longer strong, bring your attention back to your breath or whatever else is obvious in the present moment.

If a thought or image comes to your awareness, acknowledge its presence as you continue breathing. Many times thoughts remain in the background and you can be aware of them coming and going like clouds in a sky. If you get lost in thinking, once you notice the lapse in awareness, gently return to the breath. However, if a thought is obsessive and keeps coming back, bring your full attention to it and allow your breath to fade into the background. Label the type of thought, such as worry, planning, or judgmental. Check in to the body and see if there are any emotions or body sensations as well. When ready, return to the breath.

You may also notice other things, maybe a general state of energy, your alertness level, an attitude or mood. Investigate each experience until you are ready to notice the next one. Continue this in silence with your awareness open and receptive.

[*Pause.*]

Continue practicing choiceless awareness. Don't hold on to anything or make anything happen. Don't try to push anything away. Simply relax and open, allowing what is unfolding and bringing a precise and kind-hearted awareness to the flow of experience . . . look, listen, and feel as deeply as you can. Connecting with the experience and letting it go on its own accord.

[*Pause.*]

As we end, give yourself appreciation for sitting through this practice of awareness. Extend loving-kindness to yourself and wish yourself well. May I be happy, may I be safe, may I be healthy and live with ease. May I be present and compassionate to myself and others.

[*Pause.*]

Extend these wishes to all people. May we all be happy, may we all be safe, may we all be healthy and live with ease. May we all experience true listening and compassion in each other.

[*Ring bell.*]

WALKING MEDITATION (EXERCISE 8.3)

Now, let's silently shift from sitting to walking practice. Let's form a big circle.

Now, everybody turn a quarter turn to the left so you are facing the back of the person next to you.

Close your eyes, let your body be still and quiet, and feel your body standing. Stand with your feet together.

Feel your posture, notice your weight and if there is any tension or pain or maybe good feelings, too.

Good, now open your eyes, but avoid looking around as it can be distracting. Keep your eyes lowered, looking slightly ahead, aware of where you are going.

Ready? Let's begin. Everyone start walking slowly. Slowly lift one of your legs and begin to walk. Think "lifting and placing," "lifting and placing," or simply observe the movement without labeling.

Walk slowly, following the person in front of you. See if you can feel the sensations in your feet and legs. You can notice the sensations of your feet touching the ground or, if you prefer, the overall movement of your legs or arms or shifts in your weight. Either way stay connected to the sensations of walking.

> If you like, you can synchronize your breathing with your footsteps. For example, as you step with one foot, inhale; as you step with the other foot, exhale.
>
> If your mind wanders, gently bring your attention back to the sensations of walking.
>
> [*Pause.*]
>
> Where is your attention right now? If you need to, bring it back to the sensations in your feet or legs moving.
>
> Good, now everyone stop walking. Close your eyes. Feel your whole body. Simply notice whatever your experience is with openness, kindness, and curiosity.
>
> As we end, see if you can bring a sense of gratefulness for taking this time to practice mindfulness.
>
> [*Pause and then ring bell.*]

The MT asks the participants how it was for them to do a 30-minute practice: "What did you notice during this practice?" or "Did you notice anything different about doing the mindfulness practice for a longer period of time than usual?"

BREAK

This is approximately the midpoint in the session, where a 5- to 10-minute break is taken.

REVIEW OF COVERED MINDFULNESS PRINCIPLES

The MT reviews the main concepts covered in the training, discusses how they apply to ADHD (see Handout 8.3), and invites participants to share how they have applied the principles of MAPs to everyday life. This portion of the session should be driven primarily by participant comments, with the MT attuned to points that should be emphasized in correspondence with the main concepts covered in training, such as being fully present in the moment, letting go of maladaptive judgments, being open and curious, practicing compassion, appreciating the acceptance–change dialectic, and using mindfulness as a platform to choose the right action and engage in deliberate behavior.

BEYOND MAPs: ADHD AND MINDFULNESS RESOURCES

The MT discusses self-help resources that participants may use to continue their mindfulness practice, which can be guided by Handout 8.4. Additional ADHD resources independent of mindfulness practice are listed in Handout 8.5. The MT encourages participants to complete Handout 8.6, setting a plan for continuing mindfulness practices—formal and informal—over the next 2 weeks. In anticipation of participants' questions about their next options of a group or individual mindfulness and/or ADHD treatment, the MT should also read Chapter 5 of this manual, which is devoted to the topic of potential next steps once the MAPs for ADHD training is completed.

The MT makes a final point, that "life is a string of present moments—you can always drop into them or catch the next one. You can shift into mindful awareness anywhere and anytime."

The MT invites participants to reflect on the above point and share with the group their own insights on keeping mindfulness in their life beyond the MAPs for ADHD Program.

CLOSING CEREMONY

In this final reflection, the MT invites participants to sit in a circle and take turns sharing about their overall experience in the class and what they have learned. This can be done in a format of a "speaking council" exercise in which a "talking stick" is passed around to give everyone a chance to comment about their experience. Another playful variation often used in mindfulness-based trainings is throwing a ball of yarn across the circle from one participant to another. Each participant shares his or her reflection, and then hangs onto the string of yarn while throwing the ball to another person. This creates "a web of yarn" where everyone who shared a reflection is holding onto the unraveling yarn. The created web is a metaphor for interconnectedness, and the MT can reflect on how participants (and humans, in general) are all connected by common struggles and desires. After everyone shares, scissors are passed around and each person takes a piece of yarn as a reminder of the class. The yarn can be used to make a string bracelet that is worn as a tangible reminder of the mindfulness practice. These are just two ideas; MTs can come up with their own way to facilitate the final reflection.

The MT expresses appreciation for everyone in the class. A final loving-kindness meditation (loving-kindness to self, everybody in the class, and beyond) may be used to close this session.

LOVING-KINDNESS MEDITATION (EXERCISE 8.4)

Close your eyes.

[*Ring bell.*]

Take a moment and offer yourself loving-kindness for making the time to be in this class, to practice mindfulness and take care of yourself. Say to yourself "may I be happy, may I be safe, may I be healthy and live with ease."

[*Pause.*]

Next, take a moment to appreciate everyone's presence and sharing throughout the course.

Silently, wish everyone well by saying "May you be happy, may you be safe, may you be healthy and live with ease."

[*Pause.*]

Finally, think of others in your life, your loved ones, acquaintances, and all people that you may come in contact in the course of your life. See if you can extend the wishes of kindness to everyone: "May all be happy, may all be safe, may all be healthy and live with ease."

As we end, allow yourself to fully experience the feeling of kindness and gratefulness and set the intention to connect with the positive emotions in your life outside of this course.

[*Ring bell.*]

PART III

BEYOND INITIAL MAPs FOR ADHD

The End May Be Just the Beginning

In Part III of the book, we discuss the place of mindfulness-based treatment among the other commonly used treatments for adult ADHD. We outline the possible next steps after the initial MAPs for ADHD training is finished and offer treatment consideration for different clinical contexts.

CHAPTER 5

Considerations of Next Steps

In this chapter, we provide guidance on treatment considerations after the initial MAPs for ADHD Program is finished and suggestions for how to continue MAPs training beyond the eight-session protocol. Topics we cover include assessment factors, such as why some participants may need more treatment (e.g., inadequate improvement in treatment targets and other treatment goals that emerge), considerations for transitioning into individual therapy, and additional referrals guided by individualized patient goals. We also look at factors that are relevant to continuing MBI training in one form or another, such as the frequency of additional MAPs sessions, member composition, blending mindfulness content with other topics, transitioning to MAPs for special populations or peer-led groups, and including other MBI approaches. Figure 5.1 provides a quick overview of the options discussed below.

Our hope is that this chapter conveys two key messages: that mindfulness learning is often an ongoing process and that it can be combined with, and perhaps strengthened by, other treatments.

Mindfulness learning often doesn't end with MAPs. The learning can continue in different formats and/or be combined with other treatments.

WHAT DO WE DO ONCE THE INITIAL MAPs FOR ADHD GROUP IS DONE?

Now that you've reached the end of MAPs, a common question from MTs and participants alike is "Now what?" or "How do I continue this work?" A number of scenarios may play out for those who complete the group. The next steps also depend on the MT's professional background or parameters for offering the MAPs training. The MT may be offering the group only to his or her own patient panel, or the group may be open to patients in the community who may or may not be engaged with another clinician or therapist who is treating their ADHD. In the latter situation—when many participants

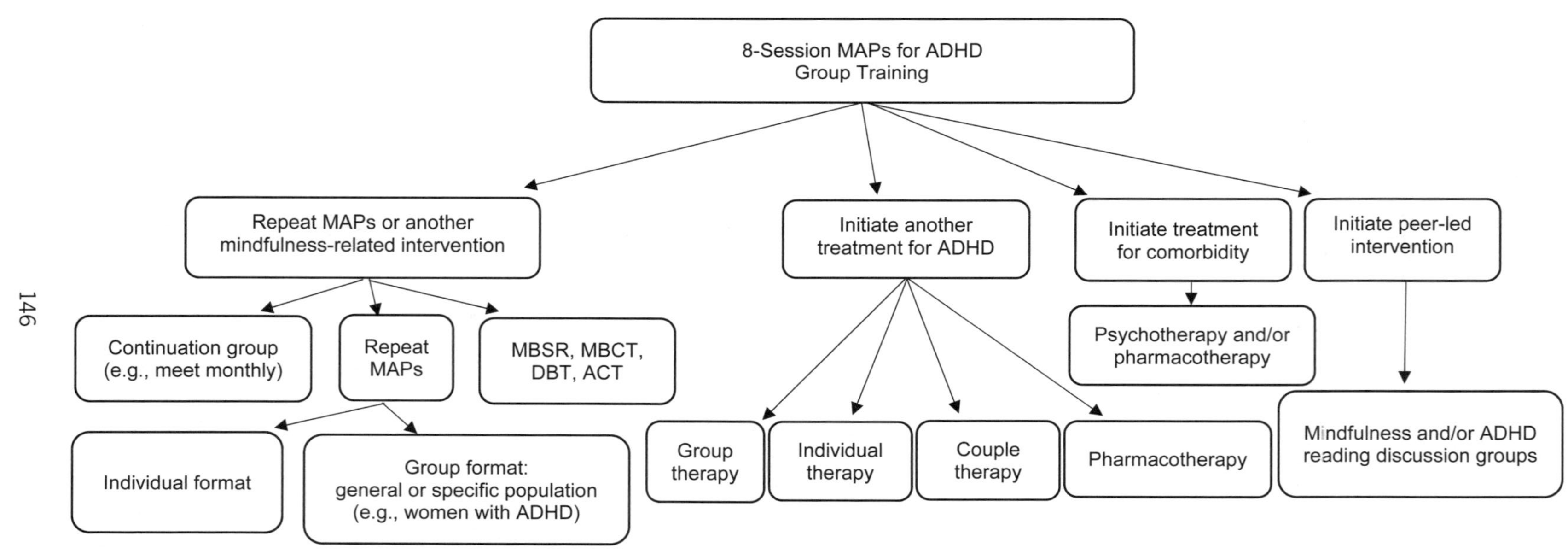

FIGURE 5.1. Flowchart of treatment options post-MAPs for adult patients with ADHD.

have other clinicians involved—the MT can offer general ideas and resources for continuation of ADHD and/or mindfulness-based treatment. These can be further pursued by the participant and their regular clinician. Or, if a participant has gotten better over the course of treatment, he or she may be ready to wrap things up and use additional self-care resources, such as mindfulness apps.

In cases where the participant wants to continue working with the MT, additional considerations arise. For example, there are cases where treatment goals have been met, but the participants want ongoing support to maintain those gains. There are cases where participants have met their treatment goals, but they have moved on to new treatment goals. Another possibility is participants who haven't met their goals, which can be for a number of reasons (e.g., poor adherence to the formal practices or extenuating life circumstances made it difficult to attend each session) and they want to continue to receive help. These scenarios and many others will emerge. There is little research to provide guidance on how to best help adults with ADHD after completing the initial MBI. However, good clinical practice informed by clear treatment goals and ways to operationalize whether treatment is working (or not) can be our reference point and guide.

DETERMINING CONTINUATION OF TREATMENT WITH MT

Individual *assessment* either through an interview or the use of symptom rating scales and questionnaires is key to determining how to move forward. Unfortunately there's no roadmap or formula that can tell MTs what to do next. Until the research starts to address "what" to do "for whom" after completing MAPs, the default should be reevaluating an individual group member's own personal goals. We provide some considerations to guide these assessments in this subsection. Many of the scenarios below are not mutually exclusive. For example, given the choice between transitioning to individual therapy or to group therapy, a potential third option is individual therapy *and* group therapy.

One area MTs may want to start with in discussing options with participants is *what to target in the next stage of treatment*. This type of discussion is individualized and we do not recommend it during a MAPs session. In terms of when this dialogue occurs, it depends on whether a group member is an ongoing patient. In those cases, the discussion would occur during an individual appointment at the conclusion of the eight-session MAPs protocol. In other cases, the discussion could occur during individual follow-up appointments MTs have with interested participants to help with referrals and treatment continuation.

During the individual session, the MT should determine if the next step will focus on targeting ADHD symptoms and related impairment, nondefining features commonly implicated in ADHD (e.g., problems with emotion regulation or self-esteem), or another psychiatric disorder. Regarding the latter, given that comorbidity is more the norm than the exception for ADHD, clinicians should be prepared for this scenario. If a particular disorder is identified, resources like the American Psychological Association's Division 12 list of empirically supported psychosocial treatments for different forms of adult psychopathology may be helpful to review (*www.div12.org/psychological-treatments*). The patient may also need a psychiatric referral for further assessment and medical treatment. Questions about whether to continue treatment with the MT or if a referral is necessary, as well as other logistical issues and preferences, may also need to be clarified.

If the focus of ongoing treatment includes ADHD, then MTs will want to clarify the treatment targets for the next phase of working together. For some adults with ADHD, *treatment success* may be defined as maintaining treatment gains and being focused on preventing a "relapse" into old ADHD behaviors. For others, it may be to attain gains that have yet to be realized. The conversation about what will constitute ongoing treatment success may be aided by the use of data that has already been collected (see Chapter 3 for suggested questionnaires). For example, have ADHD or executive function symptoms improved over the course of MAPs, such as being below a certain severity score or symptom count? If so, perhaps treatment success might be met by keeping those scores relatively stable into the next phase of treatment. If symptoms haven't improved enough, then perhaps the goal of treatment should be further symptom reduction with mindfulness-based approaches, other forms of psychotherapy, lifestyle interventions, or pharmacotherapy. Of course, the symptoms to be measured and the desired quantified values may vary on a case-by-case basis.

As the definition of what's being targeted in treatment and what success might look like becomes clearer, another consideration is *what kind of therapy setting* should be considered. The group therapy format will be most recent and therefore likely more familiar to the patient. There are benefits to group therapy that cannot be imitated in individual therapy, such as opportunities to relate to other participants and learn from them. However, individual therapy offers more individualized attention and therefore allows for a "deeper dive" into one's own particular situation, especially any trauma history, low self-esteem, addictive behaviors, and relationship issues. Of course, as we mention above, this need not be mutually exclusive; however, we caution clinicians to consider therapy fatigue, where an individual has spent so much time in therapy that they get burnt out, much like an employee may get burnt out performing the same task over and over. If an individual *and* a group component are desired, one noteworthy alternative is DBT, which has both group and individual components and could be especially useful for patients struggling with significant emotional dysregulation typical in borderline personality disorder.

In choosing *what treatment* should be adopted, the decision will often be whether or not to continue with approaches that emphasize mindfulness—another round of MAPs; related MBIs such as MBCT or MBSR, DBT, or ACT; or a community mindfulness group—versus CBT or pharmacotherapy. CBT has been shown to outperform active treatment comparison conditions in RCTs (Safren, Sprich, Mimiaga, et al., 2010; Solanto et al., 2010) and is therefore a viable empirically supported treatment option. Pharmacotherapy, particularly stimulant medications, are an established treatment for adult ADHD (Cortese et al., 2018; De Crescenzo et al., 2017) and should be discussed. While some MTs may not be licensed to provide pharmacological treatment for ADHD, they can help participants identify providers in their community for a consultation about medication options. We also list couple therapy as an option under ADHD treatments. Although there are no published treatment manuals for couple therapy and the treatment literature is small, it is promising (Wymbs & Molina, 2015), and there are some books written for clinicians (e.g., Pera & Robin, 2016) and couples (e.g., Orlov & Kohlenberger, 2014) that can provide guidance. Overall, clinicians should provide

TABLE 5.1. Treatment Continuation Factors for MTs to Consider Post-MAPs

- What to target in the next stage of treatment?
- What is considered "treatment success" or "improvement" in the next stage of treatment?
- What kind of therapy setting (e.g., individual or group) should be considered?
- What specific treatment(s) should be adopted?
- If continuing mindfulness group training, what kind of balance should there be in the next stage between the top-down direction MTs can provide and bottom-up control of the group by participants?

psychoeducation about all available treatments and work collaboratively with the individual to choose the right path for them.

Table 5.1 provides a summary of these factors involved in the decision-making process.

CONTINUATION WITH MINDFULNESS-BASED APPROACHES

If the adult with ADHD chooses to continue with a mindfulness-based approach, here are additional considerations. As there is a void of research-based recommendations at this time, we provide these options based on our clinical experience.

Frequency of Extra Sessions

Frequently, as we reach the end of the MAPS for ADHD Program, participants ask if the group can be extended. In our experience, this typically results in one more "booster" group session about 3–4 weeks after Session 8. This amount of time between the end of the MAPs for ADHD Program and the booster session is usually long enough for participants to have successes and challenges, but short enough so that those occurrences are still fresh on their minds. This duration between sessions tends to be the most optimal because, in our experience, enthusiasm seems to be high among participants—maybe because this is viewed as their "last chance" to attend group. We typically find that attendance begins to drop off for future "booster" sessions unless there is special group cohesion. This can be enhanced by considering group member composition, which we address next.

Group Member Composition for Extra Sessions

When considering future group sessions, it is important to reflect on who will be considered a group member for those sessions. While the same participants who attended the first eight sessions of MAPs for ADHD Program will likely be the only people invited to attend a "booster" session, sessions that continue on a weekly or monthly basis might be open to any ADHD individuals who have previously completed MAPs or another MBI. Such an open arrangement might impact how the group interacts—any group cohesiveness developed with other individuals in the first eight sessions will not automatically transition into a group that contains new members. However, this might be an opportunity for participants to be flexible and expand a potential support network with other adults diagnosed with ADHD.

As opposed to opening follow-up sessions to anyone who completed mindfulness training in the past, MTs might also consider narrowing the focus of who attends. We sometimes receive inquiries about female-only and college student–only groups. Such groups might be able to address situations that are more relevant for participants who share more common struggles. Indeed, one of the writers once had, quite by accident, a male-only group. The group ended up being very cohesive and more supportive than other groups.

Content for Extra Sessions

Content of the extra sessions might depend on how many extra sessions are held. If an 8-week group extends by a session or two, the content is typically focused on review of techniques previously introduced and ways to further solidify ongoing implementation of formal and informal mindfulness practices. In those cases, the sessions may be modifications of MAPs' Session 8. Discussion of online resources (e.g., *www.facebook.com/MindfulnessADHD*) and magazines (e.g., *ADDitude* magazine), joining ADHD advocacy groups (e.g., Children and Adults with Attention-Deficit/Hyperactivity Disorder [CHADD]), or reading "self-help" books devoted to the topic of ADHD may be a way to review aspects of ADHD already discussed in MAPs in a new and engaging way. Ways to maintain a regular mindfulness practice—joining other groups that practice meditation (e.g., *www.meetup.com*) or smartphone applications (e.g., CALM; Headspace; Stop, Breathe & Think)—can also be discussed. For smartphone applications, time devoted to a discussion of similarities and differences between practices taught via a particular application may be helpful. MTs may want to elicit group member involvement in this, such as having participants select different smartphone applications to pilot in between sessions, then "report back" to the group the following session.

If an 8-week group extends beyond a few sessions, should the content of sessions be a repeat of MAPs, an introduction of other non-MAPs mindfulness lessons, a shift to another treatment like CBT, or an integration of more cognitive therapy techniques within MAPs? At this time there is no research evidence to guide this decision and MTs can decide based on their clinical skills and the participants' preference.

Here, the MT may want to consider *what kind of balance* there should be in the next stage of treatment between the top-down direction MTs can provide and bottom-up control of the group by participants. For example, at the start of MAPs for ADHD when participants were new to the group, even as flexibility was modeled, group rules were set by MT. Now that those in the continuation group are MAPs "graduates," MTs might want to ask participants to decide the rules or topics for the group. MTs might ask participants what else should change about the structure or duration or frequency of the group. MTs might ask participants to suggest topics for discussion or to "vote" on topics presented (such as topics guided by CBT for adult ADHD). By doing this, MTs are encouraging and empowering adults with ADHD to take ownership of the continuation groups and to adapt the groups to their needs.

Peer-Led Option

For participants who have made sufficient progress and would prefer greater autonomy than a typical therapy setting, a peer-led group may be another option. Based on our own clinical experience, we are aware that some adults with ADHD start these kinds of groups using online resources, such as *www.meetup.com*. Resources shared at the end of Session 8 can help guide such groups in their mindfulness and/or ADHD focus.

Other MBIs

One option to highlight is that MAPs graduates may be interested in exploring alternative ways to learn mindfulness and deepening their exposure to mindfulness skills apart from an ADHD focus. Local and national resources for approaches such as MBCT, MBSR, community mindful meditation centers, and other online resources and communities can be offered by the MTs to support such interest. Modified MBCT, especially if ADHD education is included, has growing evidence that it is feasible, acceptable, and efficacious for adults with ADHD (see Chapter 2). MBSR, with its focus on stress and pain, is often suited for those struggling with such issues. While the classic MBSR groups often have 45-minute silent mindfulness practice as part of their at-home practice requirement, many MBSR instructors have modified that requirement for a shorter at-home practice (e.g., 15–30 minutes), which is likely more feasible for those with ADHD. For patients interested in blending their spiritual beliefs and mindfulness practice, groups offered at Buddhist, Christian, or other religious centers can be attractive options. Others may want to continue their practice via yoga, tai chi, or classes with a mindful activity focus, such as mindful coloring, mindful eating, or mindful photography. We recommend that MTs help participants find their own unique ways of keeping mindful awareness a part of their lives and help them maintain an attitude of curiosity about what works and what does not work for them.

We have found that it is important to acknowledge that continuing practice is difficult, and to help patients develop acceptance and self-compassion about the fact that they may not be able to do mindfulness regularly. Sayings such as "Begin again" or "Every day is a new day" can help patients feel less guilty about "dropping the ball" if they stop practicing mindfulness and can help them focus on "picking up the ball again." The MTs may choose to give patients permission to altogether forgo attempts at daily formal practice and instead focus on brief informal practice and/or occasional structured retreat or class experiences as a feasible way to keep mindfulness in their lives.

CONCLUSION

This chapter provides some considerations for MTs as they guide their participants after the initial MAPs is completed. We also want MTs to approach MAPs post Session 8 as a treatment that can grow and be adapted to meet the needs of those seeking help for their ADHD. In fact, as MTs become more and more seasoned with the MAPs guiding structure and principles, the specific practices can be tweaked and modified. For example, one of our colleagues, Dr. Lee Freedman, has used the MAPs for ADHD session structure and themes to create a mindfulness training using camera and photography exercises. We encourage MTs to build on their own strengths and make their own modifications: be open, curious, and creative. And remember that this is all in the service of helping those with ADHD come to accept and appreciate themselves, have skills to manage their ADHD, and live well.

APPENDIX

SESSION SUMMARIES AND SESSION HANDOUTS

SESSION SUMMARY FOR SESSION 1

Introduction to ADHD and Mindfulness: Reframing of ADHD

SESSION OUTLINE

1) Welcome and introductions
    - General orientation to a group setting and rules of confidentiality
    - "Getting to Know You" activity
    - Short reflection on motivation to be in the class
    - Group structure and format overview
2) ADHD introduction
    - Sharing about living with ADHD
    - ADHD psychoeducation and reframing assumptions about ADHD
3) Break
4) Mindfulness introduction
    - Definition of mindfulness and how it can help manage ADHD
    - Treatment outcome research on ADHD and mindfulness
    - Introduction to attention and the five senses: Playing with Visual Attention and Awareness (*Exercise 1.1*) and Mindful Eating (*Exercise 1.2*)
    - Sitting meditation introduction and Mindfulness of Breath (5 minutes) (*Exercise 1.3*)
5) Closing
    - Discussion of Home Practice

HOME PRACTICE

1) Formal mindfulness practice: Mindfulness of Breath (5 minutes per day)
2) Informal mindfulness practice:
    - Mindfulness of a routine daily activity, such as eating, showering, or brushing teeth
    - Brief mindful check-ins: "telephone breath" or "red light breath"

SESSION SUMMARY FOR SESSION 2

Mindful Awareness of ADHD Patterns: "What Is My ADHD Like?"

SESSION OUTLINE

1) Brief opening meditation exercise: Counting Meditation (*Exercise 2.1*)
2) Review
    - Content of previous session
    - At-Home Practice experiences
3) Session theme: Common difficulties in practicing mindful awareness
    - Introduce the acceptance–change dialectic
4) Brief meditation exercise: Mindfulness of Breath (5 minutes) (*Exercise 2.2*)
5) Break
6) Mindfulness of movement
    - Mindful Standing and Balancing (*Exercise 2.3*)
    - Mindfulness of Walking (10 minutes) (*Exercise 2.4*)
7) Closing
    - Discussion of Home Practice
    - Brief Appreciation Meditation (*Exercise 2.5*)

HOME PRACTICE

1) Formal mindfulness practice: Mindfulness of Breath (5 minutes per day). Use optional Handout 2.1 to record noted difficulties and come up with potential solutions.
2) Informal mindfulness practice:
    - Noticing one's own ADHD symptoms with curiosity

SESSION SUMMARY FOR SESSION 3

Mindful Awareness of Sound, Breath, and Body

SESSION OUTLINE

1) Brief opening meditation exercise: Mindfulness of Breath (*Exercise 3.1*)
2) Review
   - Content of previous session
   - At-Home Practice experiences
3) Session theme: Noticing shifts in attention and body awareness
4) Mindful Awareness of Music (*Exercise 3.2*)
5) Mindfulness of Sound (*Exercise 3.3*)
6) Mindful Standing and Stretching (*Exercise 3.4*)
7) Break
8) Mindfulness of Sound, Breath, and Body (*Exercise 3.5*)
9) S.T.O.P. Introduction and Practice (*Exercise 3.6*)
10) Closing
    - Discussion of Home Practice
    - Brief Appreciation Meditation (*Exercise 3.7*)

HOME PRACTICE

1) Formal mindfulness practice: Mindfulness of Sound, Breath, and Body (10 minutes per day)
2) Informal mindfulness practice:
   - Sound and walking or S.T.O.P. practice
   - Attention check-in: "Where is my attention right now?," "What am I doing right now?," and using visual reminders

SESSION SUMMARY FOR SESSION 4

Mindful Awareness of Body Sensations

SESSION OUTLINE

1) Brief opening meditation exercise: Sound, Breath, and Body (*Exercise 4.1*)
2) Review
   - Content of previous session
   - At-Home Practice experiences
3) Session theme: Being in the body
4) Body Scan (*Exercise 4.2*)
5) Break
6) Working with Pain and Discomfort (*Exercise 4.3*)
7) Mindfulness in daily life: Shoe Tying (*Exercise 4.4*)
8) Closing
   - Discussion of Home Practice
   - Brief Appreciation Meditation (*Exercise 4.5*)

HOME PRACTICE

1) Formal mindfulness practice: Sound, Breath, and Body (10 minutes per day)
2) Informal mindfulness practice:
   - Choosing a problematic ADHD-related activity (e.g., placement of keys)
   - Noticing your own ADHD symptoms with curiosity

SESSION SUMMARY FOR SESSION 5

Mindful Awareness of Thoughts

SESSION OUTLINE

1) Brief opening meditation exercise: Body Scan (*Exercise 5.1*)
2) Review
   - Content of previous session
   - At-Home Practice experiences
3) Session theme: Mindful awareness of thoughts
4) Mindfulness of Thoughts (*Exercise 5.2*)
5) Break
6) Walking with Your Thoughts (*Exercise 5.3*)
7) ADHD and judgmental thoughts
8) Sharing Experiences with Judgmental Thoughts (*Exercise 5.4*)
9) Other out-of-balance thinking
10) Self-talk as a guide
11) Closing
    - Discussion of Home Practice
    - Brief Appreciation Meditation (*Exercise 5.5*)

HOME PRACTICE

1) Formal mindfulness practice: Mindfulness of Thoughts (10 minutes per day)
2) Informal mindfulness practice:
   - Daily tracking of judgmental thoughts
   - Noticing your own ADHD symptoms with curiosity

SESSION SUMMARY FOR SESSION 6

Mindful Awareness of Emotions

SESSION OUTLINE

1) Brief opening meditation exercise: Mindfulness of Thoughts (*Exercise 6.1*)
2) Review
   - Content of previous session
   - At-Home Practice experiences
3) Session theme: Mindful awareness of emotions
4) R.A.I.N. Introduction and Practice (*Exercise 6.2*)
5) Break
6) Walking meditation: Walking with Your Emotions (*Exercise 6.3*)
7) Cultivating positive emotions: Loving-Kindness (*Exercise 6.4*)
8) Closing
   - Discussion of Home Practice
   - Brief Appreciation Meditation (*Exercise 6.6*)

HOME PRACTICE

1) Formal mindfulness practice: Loving-Kindness or the R.A.I.N. exercise (15-minutes per day). Alternatively, one can also use the Walking with Your Emotions exercise.
2) Informal mindfulness practice:
   - Practicing brief informal R.A.I.N., Loving-Kindness, or Walking with Your Emotions exercises in the course of daily life.
   - Seeing how emotions come up in different situations. This can be done using the Pleasant, Unpleasant, or Neutral Events Calendar or when tracking one's ADHD patterns.

SESSION SUMMARY FOR SESSION 7

Mindful Awareness of Presence and Interactions

SESSION OUTLINE

1) Brief opening meditation exercise: R.A.I.N. (*Exercise 7.1*)
2) Review
   - Content of previous session
   - At-Home Practice experiences
3) Session theme: Mindful awareness of presence and interactions
4) Mindful Presence Introduction and Practice (*Exercise 7.2*)
5) Discussion of different facets of attention and single-focus attention versus receptive attention
6) Break
7) Short Walking Meditation (*Exercise 7.3*)
8) Mindful awareness of interactions
9) Mindful Listening and Speaking (*Exercise 7.4*)
10) Closing
    - Discussion of Home Practice
    - Brief Appreciation Meditation (*Exercise 7.5*)

HOME PRACTICE

1) Formal mindfulness practice: Daily 15-minute sitting meditation: Mindful Presence
2) Informal mindfulness practice:
   - Mindful speaking and listening with a spouse or a friend
   - Listening mindfully during regular conversation in daily life
   - Noticing with curiosity interactions with other people

SUMMARY FOR SESSION 8

Mindful Awareness as a Life Journey

SESSION OUTLINE

1) Brief opening meditation exercise: S.T.O.P. (*Exercise 8.1*)
2) Review
   - Content of previous session
   - At-Home Practice experiences
3) Session theme: Mindful awareness as a life journey
4) Mindful Presence (*Exercise 8.2*) and Walking Meditation (*Exercise 8.3*)
5) Break
6) Review of covered mindfulness principles
7) Beyond MAPs: ADHD and mindfulness resources
8) Closing Ceremony (*Exercise 8.4*)

HANDOUT 1.1

Group Rules

Instructions: Here you may make any notes on the group rules discussed today. Some suggested areas are listed, although a few are completely blank for any rules that are unique for your group.

1. Logistics (group dates, times, and location): ____________________

   ____

2. Confidentiality: ____________________

   ____

3. Group interactions outside of group: ____________________

   ____

4. Disruptive in-session behaviors (e.g., talking too much or lateness): ____________________

   ____

5. Sharing in group: ____________________

   ____

6. ____________________

   ____

7. ____________________

   ____

8. ____________________

   ____

9. ____________________

   ____

10. ____________________

    ____

HANDOUT 1.2

What Is Mindfulness?

Mindfulness means paying attention in a particular way:
on purpose, in the present moment, and nonjudgmentally.

—*Jon Kabat-Zinn*

Two Steps of Mindfulness Practice:

1) ATTENTION
2) ATTITUDE

Instructions: Jot down some notes or draw in the area below to elaborate on what you think of when you ask yourself, "What is mindfulness?"

HANDOUT 1.3

Automatic Pilot

When we are in "automatic pilot" mode, we are not stopping to see what's going on around or inside of us. Instead, we are acting without awareness of what we are doing and what the consequences will be. This is the opposite of being mindfully aware. Being in "automatic pilot" mode often involves acting out of habit.

Instructions: Think about a time recently that you acted in "automatic pilot" mode. Use the example below to guide one of your own. If you're having difficulty coming up with an example, think about your own ADHD behaviors (e.g., times that you made a careless mistake, got lost in a conversation, lost something, procrastinated, got frustrated waiting, interrupted others, or did something impulsive). Decide ahead of time how often you will complete this form over the next week so that you have enough handouts.

Here's an example of how "automatic pilot" mode may unfold for someone with ADHD:

Situation		"Automatic Pilot" Response
At work. You decide to write that email to your coworker you've been putting off, but then your phone vibrates to indicate someone just sent you a text message.	→	Check the text message and start talking with your friend. After 10 minutes your computer "goes to sleep" and you don't know where the time has gone.

Now complete an example for yourself:

Situation		"Automatic Pilot" Response
	→	

HANDOUT 1.4

Session 1 Home Practice Sheet

Date started: ____________________

Instructions: Use this sheet to track your formal and informal practices this week.

Formal practice: 5 minutes of the Mindfulness of Breath exercise.

Informal practice:

1. Noticing the five senses in daily life. Here are some examples, though feel free to create your own:
   - Eating: Tune into the five senses for a few minutes each day. This is like the raisin exercise.
   - Showering: Notice the warmth or coolness of the water or the smell of the soap. Notice how you start: Shampoo first? Work from the top to bottom? Bottom to top? Be an observer of what you might otherwise do by habit and while on automatic pilot.
2. Brief mindful check-ins: Examples might include the "telephone breath" or "red-light breath."

Day/Date	Formal Practice How many minutes did you practice?	Informal Practice What did you do?	Comments

HANDOUT 2.1

Formal Meditation Difficulties and Solutions

Instructions: Use this sheet to help you track difficulties that emerge while engaging in formal meditation and come up with potential solutions.

STEP 1: IDENTIFY THE DIFFICULTY

It is common to experience challenges during your meditation exercises that can interfere with your regular practice. Some common examples are listed below. Circle the ones that have come up for you during meditation practice.

- Sleepiness or a lack of energy
- Restlessness or worry
- Wanting or grasping to change
- Aversion or pushing away certain experiences
- Doubt or questioning
- Distraction
- Forgetfulness
- Other: ______________________________

Now that you've named it, let's move on to the next step.

STEP 2: APPROACH THE DIFFICULTY

Now that you've identified the difficulties that you're experiencing, let's see if we can approach them in a different way. After all, difficulties are just one kind of experience that you can bring your attention and curiosity toward. Here's how you might accomplish this in the course of meditation practice:

- When you notice a difficulty, can you use words to describe your experience as though you are an observer? We call this a "witness stance," where you may say to yourself, "Oh, there is sleepiness," or "There is doubt."
- Can you investigate the challenge a bit more? What do you notice in your body? For example, how does restlessness feel inside your body? Do you notice any thoughts or judgments about the experience of restlessness? Do you notice any emotions or urges that accompany feeling restless?
- Can you keep noticing and accepting this difficulty as a part of the overall experience of trying something new like meditation? Can you let go of the struggle to rid yourself of this experience and let it be? It may change over time. In other words, can you say to yourself, "It is what it is" and not need to change the unpleasant experience but observe it (this is an acceptance-oriented solution).

(continued)

- As you notice the difficulty, you can also choose a mindful action to help relieve it. For example, if restlessness is significant, you can try breathing more deeply, shifting slowly in your seat and/or inviting your muscles to relax more. Or you can decide that instead of sitting practice you will do a mindful movement practice (this is a change-oriented solution).

Now you're ready to identify solutions more formally in Step 3.

STEP 3: IDENTIFY SOLUTIONS

Instructions: Based on the group discussion and the steps above, list out all difficulties you have experienced during the formal mindfulness meditation exercises this week. In the column next to that, list out some ideas about how you can approach these difficulties in the week ahead—these solutions may be change-oriented or may be acceptance-oriented.

Difficulties	Solution

HANDOUT 2.2

Session 2 Home Practice Sheet

Date started: ____________________

Instructions: Use this sheet to track your formal and informal practices this week.

Formal practice: 5 minutes of the Mindfulness of Breath exercise. Track difficulties that emerge during meditation by writing them down in the Comments column or use Handout 2.1.

Informal practice: Observe your own ADHD symptoms with curiosity in daily life (you can also use Handout 2.3).

Day/Date	Formal Practice How many minutes did you practice?	Informal Practice What did you do?	Comments

HANDOUT 2.3 (OPTIONAL)

Automatic Pilot

When we are in "automatic pilot" mode, we are not stopping to see what's going on around us or inside of us. Instead, we are acting without awareness of what we are doing or feeling and what the consequences will be—this is the opposite of being mindfully aware. Being on "automatic pilot" involves acting out of habit.

Instructions: Think about a time recently that you acted in "automatic pilot" mode <u>and how this is associated with ADHD for you</u>. If you can recall, also write what body sensations, thoughts, and feelings you noticed around the time of the experience. As the sessions progress, we will elaborate more on each box. This sheet can be used each week of MAPs and we recommend you make extra copies of this handout.

Day: ______________________

<u>Situation</u>	→	<u>"Automatic Pilot" Response</u>	→	<u>How is this associated with ADHD?</u>
				↓
<u>What emotions were present?</u>	←	<u>What thoughts were present?</u>	←	<u>What did you notice in your body?</u>

HANDOUT 3.1

The S.T.O.P. Practice

Instructions: Use this sheet as a visual reminder of how to do the S.T.O.P. Practice, which is a brief mindful check-in you can do in the course of your day. Post this in an area that you are likely to see repeatedly, such as on your refrigerator or by your desk.

THE S.T.O.P. PRACTICE

S = STOP

T = TAKE A BREATH

O = OBSERVE

Mindfully coach yourself to observe in the present moment without being judgmental:

> *Where is my Attention right now?*
> *Let me bring my attention to the present moment. I start by noticing Sound, Breath, or Body.*
> *What Thoughts, Emotions, or Actions do I notice right now?*

P = PROCEED

> *Do I keep going as before or do I change something?*

HANDOUT 3.2

Session 3 Home Practice Sheet

Date started: ______________________

Instructions: Use this sheet to track your formal and informal practices this week.

Formal practice: 10 minutes of the Mindfulness of Sound, Breath, and Body exercise. Continue to track difficulties that arise during your formal practice.

Informal practice:

1. Sound and walking: Identify a time in the day when you walk and for 2–3 minutes practice mindful awareness of walking.
2. Use the Attention Check-In skill daily. With this skill, use visual cues as external reminders to ask the following questions to regulate your attention: "Where is my attention right now?" and "What am I doing right now?"

Day/Date	Formal Practice How many minutes did you practice?	Informal Practice What did you do?	Comments

HANDOUT 4.1

Session 4 Home Practice Sheet

Date started: ______________________

Instructions: Use this sheet to track your formal and informal practices this week.

Formal practice: 10 minutes of the Mindfulness of Sound, Breath, and Body exercise.

Informal practice:

1. Choose a problematic ADHD-related activity involving the body (e.g., placement of keys) and practice it with mindfulness.
2. Notice your own ADHD symptoms with curiosity (you can also use Handout 2.3).

Day/Date	Formal Practice How many minutes did you practice?	Informal Practice What did you do?	Comments

HANDOUT 5.1

Session 5 Home Practice Sheet

Date started: ______________________

Instructions: Use this sheet to track your formal and informal practices this week.

Formal practice: 10 minutes of the Mind Like a Sky exercise.

Informal practice:

1. Counting the number of judgments that occur daily. An additional option is to write down thoughts that seem typical for you or are recurrent.
2. Notice your own ADHD symptoms with curiosity (you can also use Handout 2.3).

Day/Date	Formal Practice How many minutes did you practice?	Informal Practice What did you do?	Comments

HANDOUT 6.1

Aspects of Emotional Experiences

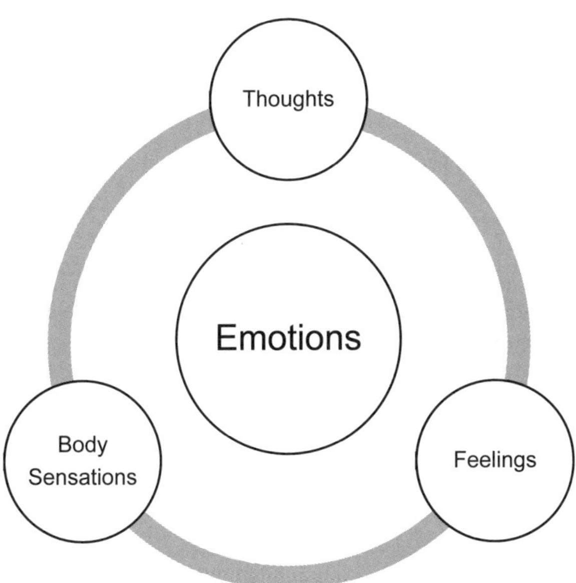

- Emotions are experiences composed of thoughts (e.g., "What a jerk!" or "I can't stand this!"), feelings (e.g., a sense of frustration or feeling overwhelmed), and body sensations (e.g., clenched teeth or neck tension).

- Positive and negative emotions are important and provide useful information. Even negative emotions can communicate something that's helpful to you!

- Emotional states are impermanent and change over time.

- Emotions are an important aspect of ADHD. In addition to feeling low self-esteem, worry, and overwhelmed, other common emotions associated with ADHD include impatience, being touchy or easily annoyed, or getting frustrated easily.

- The way adults with ADHD cope with emotions may appear helpful in the short term but may have a negative impact in the long term.

- Mindfulness can help manage emotions that are impulsive and happen quickly as well as help face emotions that are typically avoided. The intention of having what we call *brave curiosity* and self-compassion helps engage with and self-regulate emotions.

HANDOUT 6.2

Session 6 Home Practice Sheet

Date started: ______________________________

Instructions: Use this sheet to track your formal and informal practices this week.

Formal practice: 15 minutes of the Loving-Kindness exercise. You can also practice the R.A.I.N. or the Walking with Your Emotions exercise.

Informal practice:

1. Brief R.A.I.N., Loving-Kindness, or Walking with Your Emotions exercise in the course of your day, especially when emotions are stirred up.
2. See how your emotions come up in different situations. Track your reactions using Handout 2.3 or 6.4.

Day/Date	Formal Practice How many minutes did you practice?	Informal Practice What did you do?	Comments

HANDOUT 6.3

Managing Emotions with Mindfulness: The R.A.I.N. Practice

Instructions: Use this sheet as a visual reminder of how to do the R.A.I.N. practice. Post this in an area that you are likely to see repeatedly, such as on your refrigerator or by your desk.

R = Recognize
A = Accept
I = Investigate
N = Not personalize

Example:

- **R = Recognize:** Note (or label) with curiosity the feeling you are experiencing (e.g., "Oh, there is frustration").
- **A = Accept:** You don't have to like the noted feeling, but it is here—see if you can accept that the feeling is here and now.
- **I = Investigate:** To deepen your awareness, notice how the feeling is affecting your body. Notice if there are any areas of tensing muscle or how your breathing changes. As you continue to observe, see if there are any thoughts or additional feelings that may be present. Perhaps you will notice another layer of feelings, such as fear, sadness, anger, or embarrassment. Notice if there are any thoughts that go along with the feelings such as "I hate this" or self-judgments, "What's wrong with me?"
- **N = Not personalize:** Don't overly personalize or identify with the thoughts or the feelings. Remember that this is just a reaction. The reaction is like a wave that rises and eventually falls. See if you can "surf the wave" without being drowned by it.

HANDOUT 6.4

Pleasant, Unpleasant, and Neutral Events

Instructions: In this table, list one situation from each day and reflect whether the experience was pleasant, unpleasant, or neutral. In addition, write what body sensations, feelings, thoughts, and actions you observed about the experience.

Date	Situation/Experience	Was the experience pleasant, unpleasant, or neutral?	What **body sensations** did you notice?	What **feelings** did you notice?	What **thoughts** did you notice?	What **actions** did you notice?

HANDOUT 7.1

ADHD and Common Communication Pitfalls

Instructions: Below is a list of typical communication problems in ADHD that commonly occur, especially when we are in automatic pilot mode. These examples are divided into four different categories: inattention, impulsivity, executive functioning problems, and emotion dysregulation. Review these examples with a nonjudgmental attitude and identify the ones that apply to you. Then have your spouse, a family member, or a friend give you their view.

Inattention Examples	**Impulsivity Examples**	**Executive Functioning or Processing Problem Examples**	**Emotion Dysregulation Examples**
Tuning out during a conversation	Interrupting others	Going off topic or presenting in a disorganized way	Feeling intense emotions and not being able to verbally express them
Not listening or forgetting what was said	Feeling impatient during a conversation	Including too much detail in a conversation	Communicating excessive anger
Not following or feeling lost in the conversation	Talking too much, or jumping from topic to topic	Saying the same but in a different way	Being overly sensitive to criticism or rejection that may lead to quickly being defensive in communication
	Talking quickly and loudly	Extra pauses, using vocal repetitions or word fillers such as "um"	Being a "people pleaser," having trouble with conflict, difficulty saying "no" or disagreeing
	Blurting out answers or finishing others' sentences	Not finding the right word to use, using incorrect words or communicating inefficiently	Being oppositional—having trouble saying "yes" or agreeing
	Saying something you later regret (i.e., "putting your foot in your mouth")		

HANDOUT 7.2

Mindful Listening and Speaking Exercise

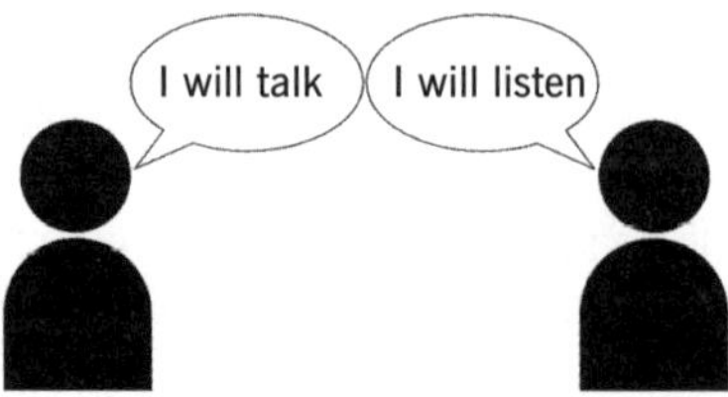

Instructions: In this exercise, you will practice speaking thoughtfully and listening fully. The exercise is done in pairs: one person is the sole speaker and the other one is the sole listener.

- Find a quiet space and sit across from your partner. Notice your posture and see if you can sit in a relaxed and receptive posture. This typically involves relaxing your face and shoulders, leaning slightly forward, avoiding crossing your arms, relaxing your hands, and keeping frequent, natural eye contact.
- Pick a topic that is meaningful for both of you and perhaps one that you have had difficulty agreeing on in the past—for example, "How can we make our household run more smoothly?"
- Have a clock or timer available so you can keep track of each turn. Take turns being the sole speaker or the sole listener for about 30 seconds before switching. Continue in this way until you exhaust the topic, up to 10 minutes. Alternatively, you can also decide to give each other 5 minutes of uninterrupted talking (or listening) before switching.
- Practice relaxed body and relaxed breathing throughout the conversation.

Guidelines for Mindful Listening

- Bring full attention to your partner and practice consistent listening. For example, if distracted or daydreaming, keep bringing your attention back to your partner as much as possible.
- Practice "receiving the information" nonjudgmentally without having to do anything else.
- Withhold any impulses to interrupt, or give feedback or join the conversation. In this exercise, practice being a quiet listener versus a listener that is offering a lot of verbal encouragement. Even well-intentioned validations, such as "Yes, I feel the same way" or "You are right," may feel to the speaker like an interruption.
- Practice to embody an open and empathetic presence.

Guidelines for Mindfully Speaking

- Bring the intention to speak a bit more slowly than usual, choosing your words thoughtfully.
- Practice "speaking from the heart," choosing to be honest, kind, and sharing your feelings. Practice using "I" statements versus describing what you think the other person is doing or should be doing.

HANDOUT 7.3

Session 7 Home Practice Sheet

Date started: ____________________

Instructions: Use this sheet to track your formal and informal practices this week.

Formal practice: 15 minutes of the Mindful Presence exercise.

Informal practice:

1. Ask a friend, family member, or spouse to do a mindfulness exercise with you. Either (1) review the ADHD and Communication Pitfalls Handout with them and get their feedback or (2) find one time to practice mindful listening and speaking with that person. See Handouts 7.1 and 7.2.
2. Listen mindfully when engaged in regular conversations with others in the course of the week. Pay attention to these interactions and consider using Handout 2.3 to reflect on your communication.
3. Pay attention to interactions and consider using optional Handout 2.3 to build on "putting things together" that were also learned in previous sessions.

Day/Date	Formal Practice How many minutes did you practice?	Informal Practice What did you do?	Comments

HANDOUT 8.1

Informal Practice Ideas

You can bring mindful awareness to anything, anytime!
Instructions: Each week, take a look at this list and pick one or two ways to keep mindfulness in your daily activities.

- Mindful eating (e.g., mindful snack or lunch)
- Mindful movement (e.g., walking, stretching, dancing, yoga)
- Taking three mindful breaths
- Showering
- Washing hands
- Checking the time (watch, clock, or cell phone)
- Browsing the internet
- Email
- Answering the telephone
- Washing dishes
- Chopping vegetables
- Preparing coffee
- Playing with your pet
- Making your bed
- Folding laundry
- Brushing teeth
- Shaving
- Driving
- Walking to the bathroom at work
- Talking with coworkers
- Talking with loved ones
- Playing with kids
- Putting kids to sleep
- Being in nature, listening to nature sounds
- Gardening
- Listening to music
- Making art or doing a creative task
- Organizing your room, desk, office
- Making a to do list or using a calendar
- S.T.O.P. reminders
- R.A.I.N. reminders

HANDOUT 8.2

Strategies for Keeping Mindfulness in Your Life

Instructions: This form lists some concrete behavioral strategies and resources you may want to use to keep your daily mindfulness routine going. Check these out and see what works for you.

- Create visual reminders of mindfulness practice (e.g., a picture frame with the word *breathe* or *now*).
- Use daily occurrences or habitual activities as a reminder to be mindful (e.g., red lights remind you to stop your car. Let them remind you to stop and breathe. Or every time you turn your computer on, make a point to do a mindful check-in, noticing sounds, then your breath, body, thoughts, and feelings).
- Set email or calendar reminders for yourself to practice.
- Use electronic organizers or calendars to schedule mindfulness practice.
- Have a friend or a spouse be your mindfulness buddy or coach.
- Attend an ongoing meditation group alone or with a family member.
- Go to a periodic mindfulness workshops or retreat.
- Use *The Mindfulness Prescription for Adult ADHD* self-help book as a course refresher or reference. Using the book, you can start your own mindfulness group (*www.meetup.com* can be helpful with getting started).
- Continue to engage in learning about ADHD and/or mindfulness via smartphone applications, websites, or books. See selected examples listed in Handouts 8.4 and 8.5.

HANDOUT 8.3

Why Use Mindfulness for ADHD?

- *Improve ADHD symptoms and related self-regulation difficulties.* ADHD is associated with difficulties in executive functioning, which can result in difficulty regulating attention, mood, and behavior. Research studies suggest that mindfulness strengthens self-regulation skills.
- *Lower stress.* Living with ADHD often comes with increased stress. Mindfulness has been shown to lower perceived stress. This practice also provides skills to shift from a stressed mind-body state to a more relaxed mind-body state through mindful breathing and other exercises in present-moment awareness.
- *Decrease risk for anxiety, depression, impulse-control problems (substance abuse, eating disorders).* ADHD is known to increase risk for such difficulties, presumably by self-regulation difficulties.
- *Increase self-acceptance and self-advocacy.* The self-compassion training of mindfulness can counteract insecurity or shame, often reported with ADHD.
- *Improve communication, which can enhance relationship with others (e.g., spouses, children, coworkers).* Mindfulness can provide a foundation for being more present to people you interact with on a regular basis. This can allow for better listening and deeper communication.

HANDOUT 8.4

Examples of Resources Related to Mindfulness and ADHD

MINDFULNESS APPS

- Mindfulness Apps—go to App Store or Google Play Store and search "mindfulness" or "meditation." Some examples include Insight Timer; Stop, Breathe & Think (SBT); Headspace; Calm

SELECTED WEBSITES

- A link to the meditations for this book can be found on The Guilford Press website (see the box at the end of the table of contents)
- *www.facebook.com/MindfulnessADHD*
- *https://mindfullyadd.com*
- *http://www.Mindful.org*—online magazine about "everything mindfulness"
- *www.marc.ucla.edu*—classes and mindfulness workshop including online offerings
- *www.umassmed.edu/cfm/index.aspx*—University of Massachusetts Center for Mindfulness, the home of MBSR
- *www.bemindful.co.uk*—a British website highlighting info about mindfulness, MBSR, and MBCT
- *https://goamra.org*—a guide to what's latest in mindfulness research

BOOKS

ADHD and Mindfulness

- *The Mindfulness Prescription for Adult ADHD* by Lidia Zylowska
- *The Family ADHD Solution: A Scientific Approach to Maximizing Your Child's Attention and Minimizing Parental Stress* or *Mindful Parenting for ADHD* by Mark Bertin
- *Connected Kids* by Lorraine Murray
- *Mindfulness for Kids with ADHD* and *Mindfulness for Teens with ADHD* by Debra Burdick
- *Living Well with ADHD* by Terry Huff

General Books on Mindfulness

- *The Mindful Child* and *Mindful Games* by Susan Kaiser-Greenland
- *Mindfulness Made Easy* by Ed Halliwell
- *Still Quiet Place* by Amy Saltzman
- *Child's Mind* by Christopher Willard
- *Mindful Movements: Ten Exercises for Well-Being* by Thich Nhat Hanh

(continued)

Examples of Resources Related to Mindfulness and ADHD *(page 2 of 2)*

- *The MBSR Workbook* by Bob Stahl and Elisha Goldstein
- *The Mindful Way Workbook* (the MBCT workbook) by John Teasdale, Mark Williams, and Zindel Segal
- *Full Catastrophe Living* by Jon Kabat-Zinn
- *Fully Present* by Susan Smalley and Diana Winston
- *The Mindful Brain* by Daniel Siegel
- *Self-Compassion* by Kristen Neff

HANDOUT 8.5

Additional ADHD Resources

SELECTED BOOKS

Barkley, R. A. (2010). *Taking charge of adult ADHD.* New York: Guilford Press.

Hallowell, E. M., & Ratey, J. J. (2011). *Driven to distraction (revised): Recognizing and coping with attention deficit disorder from childhood through adulthood.* New York: Anchor Books.

Kelly, K., & Ramundo, P. (2006). *You mean I'm not lazy, stupid or crazy?! The classic self-help book for adults with attention deficit disorder.* New York: Scribner.

Mate, G. (1999). *How attention deficit disorder originates and what you can do about it.* New York: Penguin.

Moulton Sarkis, S. (2015). *Natural relief for adult ADHD: Complementary strategies for increasing focus, attention, and motivation with or without medication.* Oakland, CA: New Harbinger.

Murphy, K. R., & Levert, S. (1995). *Out of the fog: Treatment options and coping strategies for adult attention deficit disorder.* New York: Skylight Press.

Nadeau, K. G. (1996). *Adventures in fast forward: Life, love, and work for the ADD adult.* New York: Routledge.

Orlov, M. (2010). *The ADHD effect on marriage: Understand and rebuild your relationship in six steps.* Plantation, FL: Specialty Press.

Pera, G. (2008). *Is it you, me, or adult A.D.D.? Stopping the roller coaster when someone you love has attention deficit disorder.* San Francisco: 1201 Alarm Press.

Ramsay, J. R., & Rostain, A. L. (2015). *The adult ADHD tool kit: Using CBT to facilitate coping inside and out.* New York: Routledge.

Sari, S., & Frank, M. (2019). *A radical guide for women with ADHD: Embrace neurodiversity, love boldly, and break through barriers.* Oakland, CA: New Harbinger.

Tuckman, A. (2012). *Understand your brain, get more done: The ADHD executive functions workbook.* Plantation, FL: Specialty Press.

WEBSITES FOR ADULTS WITH ADHD AND THEIR FAMILIES

ADDitude: *www.additudemag.com*

Attention Deficit Disorder Association (ADDA): *https://add.org*

Children and Adult with Attention-Deficit/Hyperactivity Disorder (CHADD): *https://chadd.org*

TotallyADD: *https://totallyadd.com*

Attention Talk Radio: *www.blogtalkradio.com/attentiontalkradio*

HANDOUT 8.6

Setting Intentions for the Next 2 Weeks

Instructions: Use this form to set an intention on how you want to keep mindfulness practices in your daily life. Take a few minutes to fill it out and list some concrete plans on what you can do in the next 2 weeks.

Why is it important to me to keep mindfulness in my life?

____

____

____

____

____

____

Formal practice ideas:

____

____

____

____

____

____

Informal practice ideas:

____

____

____

____

____

____

References

Aadil, M., Cosme, R. M., & Chernaik, J. (2017). Mindfulness-based cognitive behavioral therapy as an adjunct treatment of attention deficit hyperactivity disorder in young adults: A literature review. *Cureus, 9*(5), e1269.

Abramovitch, A., & Schweiger, A. (2009). Unwanted intrusive and worrisome thoughts in adults with attention deficit/hyperactivity disorder. *Psychiatry Research, 168*(3), 230–233.

American Psychiatric Association. (2013). *Diagnostic and statistical manual of mental disorders* (5th ed.). Arlington, VA: Author.

Bachmann, K., Lam, A. P., & Philipsen, A. (2016). Mindfulness-based cognitive therapy and the adult ADHD brain: A neuropsychotherapeutic perspective. *Frontiers in Psychiatry, 7,* 117.

Baer, R. (2016). Assessment of mindfulness and closely related constructs: Introduction to the special issue. *Psychological Assessment, 28*(7), 787–790.

Baer, R. A., Smith, G. T., Lykins, E., Button, D., Krietemeyer, J., Sauer, S., . . . Williams, J. M. (2008). Construct validity of the five facet mindfulness questionnaire in meditating and nonmeditating samples. *Assessment, 15*(3), 329–342.

Baijal, S., & Gupta, R. (2008). Meditation-based training: A possible intervention for attention deficit hyperactivity disorder. *Psychiatry (Edgmont), 5*(4), 48–55.

Barkley, R. A. (1997). Behavioral inhibition, sustained attention, and executive functions: Constructing a unifying theory of ADHD. *Psychological Bulletin, 121*(1), 65–94.

Barkley, R. A. (2010). Deficient emotional self-regulation is a core component of attention-deficit/hyperactivity disorder. *Journal of ADHD and Related Disorders, 1*(2), 5–37.

Barkley, R. A. (2011a). *Barkley Adult ADHD Rating Scale—IV (BAARS-IV).* New York: Guilford Press.

Barkley, R. A. (2011b). *The Deficits in Executive Functioning Scale (DEFS): Assessing problems in executive functioning in daily life activities.* New York: Guilford Press.

Barkley, R. A. (Ed.). (2015). *Attention-deficit/hyperactivity disorder: A handbook for diagnosis and treatment* (4th ed.). New York: Guilford Press.

Barkley, R. A., & Fischer, M. (2010). The unique contribution of emotional impulsiveness to impairment in major life activities in hyperactive children as adults. *Journal of the American Academy of Child and Adolescent Psychiatry, 49*(5), 503–513.

Barkley, R. A., & Murphy, K. R. (2006). *Attention-deficit/hyperactivity disorder: A clinical workbook* (3rd ed.). New York: Guilford Press.

Barkley, R. A., & Murphy, K. R. (2010). Deficient emotional self-regulation in adults with attention-deficit/hyperactivity disorder (ADHD): The relative contributions of emotional impulsiveness and ADHD symptoms to adaptive impairments in major life activities. *Journal of ADHD and Related Disorders, 1*(4), 5–28.

Barkley, R. A., Murphy, K. R., & Fischer, M. (2008). *ADHD in adults: What the science says.* New York: Guilford Press.

Barkley, R. A., & Peters, H. (2012). The earliest reference to ADHD in the medical literature?: Melchior Adam Weikard's description in 1775 of "attention deficit" (Mangel der Aufmerksamkeit, Attentio Volubilis). *Journal of Attention Disorders, 16*(8), 623–630.

Beck, A. T., Epstein, N., Brown, G., & Steer, R. A. (1988). An inventory for measuring clinical anxiety: Psychometric properties. *Journal of Consulting and Clinical Psychology, 56*(6), 893–897.

Beck, A. T., & Steer, R. A. (1984). Internal consistencies of the original and revised Beck Depression Inventory. *Journal of Clinical Psychology, 40*(6), 1365–1367.

Beck, A. T., Ward, C. H., Mendelson, M., Mock, J., & Erbaugh, J. (1961). An inventory for measuring depression. *Archives of General Psychiatry, 4*, 561–571.

Bishop, S. R., Lau, M., Shapiro, S., Carlson, L., Anderson, N. D., Carmody, J., . . . Devins, G. (2004). Mindfulness: A proposed operational definition. *Clinical Psychology: Science and Practice, 11*(3), 230–241.

Black, D. S. (2014). Mindfulness-based interventions: An antidote to suffering in the context of substance use, misuse, and addiction. *Substance Use and Misuse, 49*(5), 487–491.

Black, D. S., Milam, J., & Sussman, S. (2009). Sitting-meditation interventions among youth: A review of treatment efficacy. *Pediatrics, 124*(3), e532–e541.

Bodhi, B. (2011). What does mindfulness really mean?: A canonical perspective. *Contemporary Buddhism, 12*, 19–39.

Bögels, S., Hoogstad, B., van Dun, L., de Schutter, S., & Restifo, K. (2008). Mindfulness training for adolescents with externalizing disorders and their parents. *Behavioral and Cognitive Psychotherapy, 36*(2), 193–209.

Bögels, S., & Restifo, K. (2014). *Mindful parenting: A guide for mental health practitioners.* New York: Springer.

Boonstra, A. M., Oosterlaan, J., Sergeant, J. A., & Buitelaar, J. K. (2005). Executive functioning in adult ADHD: A meta-analytic review. *Psychological Medicine, 35*(8), 1097–1108.

Bowen, S., Chawla, N., & Marlatt, G. A. (2011). *Mindfulness-based relapse prevention for addictive behaviors: A clinician's guide.* New York: Guilford Press.

Bowen, S., Witkiewitz, K., Clifasefi, S. L., Grow, J., Chawla, N., Hsu, S. H., . . . Larimer, M. E. (2014). Relative efficacy of mindfulness-based relapse prevention, standard relapse prevention, and treatment as usual for substance use disorders: A randomized clinical trial. *JAMA Psychiatry, 71*(5), 547–556.

Brewer, J. A., & Garrison, K. A. (2014). The posterior cingulate cortex as a plausible mechanistic target of meditation: Findings from neuroimaging. *Annals of the New York Academy of Sciences, 1307*, 19–27.

Brewer, J. A., Worhunsky, P. D., Gray, J. R., Tang, Y. Y., Weber, J., & Kober, H. (2011). Meditation experience is associated with differences in default mode network activity and connectivity. *Proceedings of the National Academy of Sciences of the USA, 108*(50), 20254–20259.

Brown, K. W., & Ryan, R. M. (2003). The benefits of being present: Mindfulness and its role in psychological well-being. *Journal of Personality and Social Psychology, 84*(4), 822–848.

Bueno, V. F., Kozasa, E. H., da Silva, M. A., Alves, T. M., Louza, M. R., & Pompeia, S. (2015). Mindfulness meditation improves mood, quality of life, and attention in adults with attention deficit hyperactivity disorder. *BioMed Research International, 2015*, 962857.

Burdick, D. (2017). *Mindfulness for teens with ADHD: A skill-building workbook to help you focus and succeed.* Oakland, CA: New Harbinger.

Cairncross, M., & Miller, C. J. (2016). The effectiveness of mindfulness-based therapies for ADHD: A meta-analytic review. *Journal of Attention Disorders, 24*(5), 627–643.

Cassone, A. R. (2015). Mindfulness training as an adjunct to evidence-based treatment for ADHD within families. *Journal of Attention Disorders, 19*(2), 147–157.

Castellanos, F. X., Margulies, D. S., Kelly, C., Uddin, L. Q., Ghaffari, M., Kirsch, A., . . . Milham, M. P. (2008). Cingulate-precuneus interactions: A new locus of dysfunction in adult attention-deficit/hyperactivity disorder. *Biological Psychiatry, 63*(3), 332–337.

Chambers, R., Gullone, E., & Allen, N. B. (2009). Mindful emotion regulation: An integrative review. *Clinical Psychology Review, 29*(6), 560–572.

Chen, K. W., Berger, C. C., Manheimer, E., Forde, D., Magidson, J., Dachman, L., & Lejuez, C. W. (2012). Meditative therapies for reducing anxiety: A systematic review and meta-analysis of randomized controlled trials. *Depression and Anxiety, 29*(7), 545–562.

Cheung, K. K., Wong, I. C., Ip, P., Chan, P. K., Lin, C. H., Wong, L. Y., & Chan, E. W. (2015). Experiences of adolescents and young adults with ADHD in Hong Kong: Treatment services and clinical management. *BMC Psychiatry, 15*, 95.

Chiesa, A., Calati, R., & Serretti, A. (2011). Does mindfulness training improve cognitive abilities?: A systematic review of neuropsychological findings. *Clinical Psychology Review, 31*(3), 449–464.

Chiesa, A., & Malinowski, P. (2011). Mindfulness-based approaches: Are they all the same? *Journal of Clinical Psychology, 67*(4), 404–424.

Chiesa, A., & Serretti, A. (2011a). Mindfulness-based interventions for chronic pain: A systematic review of the evidence. *Journal of Alternative and Complementary Medicine, 17*(1), 83–93.

Chiesa, A., & Serretti, A. (2011b). Mindfulness based cognitive therapy for psychiatric disorders: A systematic review and meta-analysis. *Psychiatry Research, 187*(3), 441–453.

Chiesa, A., & Serretti, A. (2014). Are mindfulness-based interventions effective for substance use disorders?: A systematic review of the evidence. *Substance Use and Misuse, 49*(5), 492–512.

Christoff, K., Gordon, A. M., Smallwood, J., Smith, R., & Schooler, J. W. (2009). Experience sampling during fMRI reveals default network and executive system contributions to mind wandering. *Proceedings of the National Academy of Sciences of the USA, 106*(21), 8719–8724.

Cohen, S., Kamarck, T., & Mermelstein, R. (1983). A global measure of perceived stress. *Journal of Health and Social Behavior, 24*(4), 385–396.

Conners, C. K. (1995). *The Conners Continuous Performance Test*. Toronto: Multi-Health Systems.

Conners, C. K., Erhardt, D., & Sparrow, E. (1999). *Conners' Adult ADHD Rating Scales (CAARS) technical manual*. North Tonawanda, NY: Multi-Health Systems.

Cortese, S., Adamo, N., Del Giovane, C., Mohr-Jensen, C., Hayes, A. J., Carucci, S., . . . Cipriani, A. (2018). Comparative efficacy and tolerability of medications for attention-deficit hyperactivity disorder in children, adolescents, and adults: A systematic review and network meta-analysis. *Lancet Psychiatry, 5*(9), 727–738.

Cortese, S., Faraone, S. V., & Sergeant, J. (2011). What should be said to the lay public regarding ADHD etiology based on unbiased systematic quantitative empirical evidence. *American Journal of Medical Genetics, Part B, Neuropsychiatric Genetics, 156B*(8), 987–988.

Creswell, J. D., Taren, A. A., Lindsay, E. K., Greco, C. M., Gianaros, P. J., Fairgrieve, A., . . . Ferris, J. L. (2016). Alterations in resting state functional connectivity link mindfulness meditation with reduced interleukin-6: A randomized controlled trial. *Biological Psychiatry, 80*(1), 53–61.

Crowe, M., Jordan, J., Burrell, B., Jones, V., Gillon, D., & Harris, S. (2016). Mindfulness-based stress reduction for long-term physical conditions: A systematic review. *Australian and New Zealand Journal of Psychiatry, 50*(1), 21–32.

Cubillo, A., Halari, R., Smith, A., Taylor, E., & Rubia, K. (2012). A review of fronto-striatal and fronto-cortical brain abnormalities in children and adults with attention deficit hyperactivity disorder (ADHD) and new evidence for dysfunction in adults with ADHD during motivation and attention. *Cortex, 48*(2), 194–215.

Davidson, R. J., & Kaszniak, A. W. (2015). Conceptual and methodological issues in research on mindfulness and meditation. *American Psychologist, 70*(7), 581–592.

Davis, N. O., & Mitchell, J. T. (2020). Mindfulness meditation training for adolescents with ADHD. In S. P. Becker (Ed.), *ADHD in adolescents: Development, assessment, and treatment* (pp. 369–390). New York: Guilford Press.

De Crescenzo, F., Cortese, S., Adamo, N., & Janiri, L. (2017). Pharmacological and non-pharmacological treatment of adults with ADHD: A meta-review. *Evidence-Based Mental Health, 20*(1), 4–11.

Del Re, A. C., Fluckiger, C., Goldberg, S. B., & Hoyt, W. T. (2013). Monitoring mindfulness practice quality: An important consideration in mindfulness practice. *Psychotherapy Research, 23*(1), 54–66.

Demarzo, M. M., Montero-Marin, J., Cuijpers, P., Zabaleta-del-Olmo, E., Mahtani, K. R., Vellinga, A., . . . Garcia-Campayo, J. (2015). The efficacy of mindfulness-based interventions in primary care: A meta-analytic review. *Annals of Family Medicine, 13*(6), 573–582.

DeSole, L. (2011). Special issue: Eating disorders and mindfulness: Introduction. *Eating Disorders, 19*(1), 1–5.

Dimidjian, S., & Segal, Z. V. (2015). Prospects for a clinical science of mindfulness-based intervention. *American Psychologist, 70*(7), 593–620.

Dreyfus, G. (2011). Is mindfulness present-centred and non-judgmental?: A discussion of the cognitive dimensions of mindfulness. *Contemporary Buddhism, 12,* 41–54.

Dunne, J. (2011). Toward an understanding of non-dual mindfulness. *Contemporary Buddhism, 12,* 71–88.

Edel, M. A., Holter, T., Wassink, K., & Juckel, G. (2017). A comparison of mindfulness-based group training and skills group training in adults with ADHD. *Journal of Attention Disorders, 21*(6), 533–539.

Ellamil, M., Fox, K. C., Dixon, M. L., Pritchard, S., Todd, R. M., Thompson, E., & Christoff, K. (2016). Dynamics of neural recruitment surrounding the spontaneous arising of thoughts in experienced mindfulness practitioners. *NeuroImage, 136,* 186–196.

Evans, S., Ling, M., Hill, B., Rinehart, N., Austin, D., & Sciberras, E. (2018). Systematic review of meditation-based interventions for children with ADHD. *European Child and Adolescent Psychiatry, 27*(1), 9–27.

Fair, D. A., Posner, J., Nagel, B. J., Bathula, D., Dias, T. G., Mills, K. L., . . . Nigg, J. T. (2010). Atypical default network connectivity in youth with attention-deficit/hyperactivity disorder. *Biological Psychiatry, 68*(12), 1084–1091.

Fan, J., & Posner, M. (2004). Human attentional networks. *Psychiatrische Praxis, 31*(Suppl. 2), S210–S214.

Fjorback, L. O., Arendt, M., Ornbol, E., Fink, P., & Walach, H. (2011). Mindfulness-based stress reduction and mindfulness-based cognitive therapy: A systematic review of randomized controlled trials. *Acta Psychiatrica Scandinavica, 124*(2), 102–119.

Frazier, T. W., Youngstrom, E. A., & Naugle, R. I. (2007). The latent structure of attention-deficit/hyperactivity disorder in a clinic-referred sample. *Neuropsychology, 21*(1), 45–64.

Galante, J., Iribarren, S. J., & Pearce, P. F. (2013). Effects of mindfulness-based cognitive therapy on mental disorders: A systematic review and meta-analysis of randomised controlled trials. *Journal of Research in Nursing, 18*(2), 133–155.

Galla, B. M., O'Reilly, G. A., Kitil, M. J., Smalley, S. L., & Black, D. S. (2015). Community-based mindfulness program for disease prevention and health promotion: Targeting stress reduction. *American Journal of Health Promotion, 30*(1), 36–41.

Garland, E. L., Fredrickson, B. L., Kring, A. M., Johnson, D. P., Meyer, P. S., & Penn, D. L. (2010). Upward spirals of positive emotions counter downward spirals of negativity: Insights from the broaden-and-build theory and affective neuroscience on the treatment of emotion dysfunctions and deficits in psychopathology. *Clinical Psychology Review, 30*(7), 849–864.

Gethin, R. (2011). On some definitions of mindfulness. *Contemporary Buddhism, 12,* 263–279.

Goldstein, S., & Teeter Ellison, A. (2002). *Clinician's guide to adult ADHD: Assessment and intervention.* San Diego, CA: Academic Press.

Gotink, R. A., Chu, P., Busschbach, J. J., Benson, H., Fricchione, G. L., & Hunink, M. G. (2015). Standardised mindfulness-based interventions in healthcare: An overview of systematic reviews and meta-analyses of RCTs. *PLOS ONE, 10*(4), e0124344.

Gratz, K. L., & Roemer, L. (2004). Multidimensional assessment of emotion regulation and dysregulation: Development, factor structure, and initial validation of the Difficulties in Emotion Regulation Scale. *Journal of Psychopathology and Behavioral Assessment, 26,* 41–54.

Gratz, K. L., & Tull, M. T. (2010). Emotion regulation as a mechanism of change in acceptance- and mindfulness-based treatments. In R. A. Baer (Ed.), *Assessing mindfulness and acceptance processes in clients: Illuminating the theory and practice of change* (pp. 107–133). Oakland, CA: Context Press/New Harbinger.

Grossman, P. (2008). On measuring mindfulness in psychosomatic and psychological research. *Journal of Psychosomatic Research, 64*(4), 405–408.

Grossman, P. (2011). Defining mindfulness by how poorly I think I pay attention during everyday awareness and other intractable problems for psychology's (re)invention of mindfulness: Comment on Brown et al. (2011). *Psychological Assessment, 23*(4), 1034–1040; discussion 1041–1046.

Gu, J., Strauss, C., Bond, R., & Cavanagh, K. (2015). How do mindfulness-based cognitive therapy and mindfulness-based stress reduction improve mental health and wellbeing?: A systematic review and meta-analysis of mediation studies. *Clinical Psychology Review, 37,* 1–12.

Gu, Y., Xu, G., & Zhu, Y. (2018). A randomized controlled trial of mindfulness-based cognitive therapy for college students with ADHD. *Journal of Attention Disorders, 22*(4), 388–399.

Guendelman, S., Medeiros, S., & Rampes, H. (2017). Mindfulness and emotion regulation: Insights from neurobiological, psychological, and clinical studies. *Frontiers in Psychology, 8,* 220.

Hall, C. L., Newell, K., Taylor, J., Sayal, K., Swift, K. D., & Hollis, C. (2013). "Mind the gap"—Mapping services for young people with ADHD transitioning from child to adult mental health services. *BMC Psychiatry, 13,* 186.

Hanh, T. N. (2001). *Thich Nhat Hanh: Essential writings.* Maryknoll, NY: Orbis Books.

Harrington, A., & Dunne, J. D. (2015). When mindfulness is therapy: Ethical qualms, historical perspectives. *American Psychologist, 70*(7), 621–631.

Hasenkamp, W., Wilson-Mendenhall, C. D., Duncan, E., & Barsalou, L. W. (2012). Mind wandering and attention during focused meditation: A fine-grained temporal analysis of fluctuating cognitive states. *NeuroImage, 59*(1), 750–760.

Hayes, S. C., Follette, V. M., & Linehan, M. M. (Eds.). (2004). *Mindfulness and acceptance: Expanding the cognitive-behavioral tradition.* New York: Guilford Press.

Hayes, S. C., Luoma, J. B., Bond, F. W., Masuda, A., & Lillis, J. (2006). Acceptance and commitment therapy: Model, processes and outcomes. *Behaviour Research and Therapy, 44*(1), 1–25.

Hayes, S. C., Strosahl, K. D., & Wilson, K. G. (1999). *Acceptance and Commitment Therapy: An experiential approach to behavior change.* New York: Guilford Press.

Hayes, S. C., Strosahl, K. D., & Wilson, K. G. (2012). *Acceptance and Commitment Therapy: The process and practice of mindful change* (2nd ed.). New York: Guilford Press.

Hechtman, L., Swanson, J. M., Sibley, M. H., Stehli, A., Owens, E. B., Mitchell, J. T., . . . M. T. A. Cooperative Group. (2016). Functional adult outcomes 16 years after childhood diagnosis of attention-deficit/hyperactivity disorder: MTA results. *Journal of the American Academy of Child and Adolescent Psychiatry, 55*(11), 945–952.e2.

Hepark, S., Janssen, L., de Vries, A., Schoenberg, P. L., Donders, R., Kan, C. C., & Speckens, A. E. (2019). The efficacy of adapted MBCT on core symptoms and executive functioning in adults with ADHD: A preliminary randomized controlled trial. *Journal of Attention Disorders, 23*(4), 351–362.

Hepark, S., Kan, C. C., & Speckens, A. (2014). Feasibility and effectiveness of mindfulness training in adults with ADHD: A pilot study. *Tijdschrift voor Psychiatrie, 56*(7), 471–476.

Hervey, A. S., Epstein, J. N., & Curry, J. F. (2004). Neuropsychology of adults with attention-deficit/hyperactivity disorder: A meta-analytic review. *Neuropsychology, 18*(3), 485–503.

Hinshaw, S. P., & Ellison, K. (2015). *ADHD: What everyone needs to know.* New York: Oxford University Press.

Hofmann, S. G., Sawyer, A. T., Witt, A. A., & Oh, D. (2010). The effect of mindfulness-based therapy on anxiety and depression: A meta-analytic review. *Journal of Consulting and Clinical Psychology, 78*(2), 169–183.

Hölzel, B. K., Lazar, S. W., Gard, T., Schuman-Olivier, Z., Vago, D. R., & Ott, U. (2011). How does mindfulness meditation work?: Proposing mechanisms of action from a conceptual and neural perspective. *Perspectives on Psychological Science, 6*(6), 537–559.

Hoxhaj, E., Sadohara, C., Borel, P., D'Amelio, R., Sobanski, E., Muller, H., . . . Philipsen, A. (2018). Mindfulness vs psychoeducation in adult ADHD: A randomized controlled trial. *European Archives of Psychiatry and Clinical Neuroscience, 268*(4), 321–335.

Janssen, L., de Vries, A. M., Hepark, S., & Speckens, A. E. M. (2020). The feasibility, effectiveness, and process of change of mindfulness-based cognitive therapy for adults with ADHD: A mixed-method pilot study. *Journal of Attention Disorders, 24*(6), 928–942.

Janssen, L., Kan, C. C., Carpentier, P. J., Sizoo, B., Hepark, S., Schellekens, M. P. J., . . . Speckens, A. E. M. (2019). Mindfulness-based cognitive therapy v. treatment as usual in adults with ADHD: A multicentre, single-blind, randomised controlled trial. *Psychological Medicine, 49*(1), 55–65.

Jensen, P. S., Mrazek, D., Knapp, P. K., Steinberg, L., Pfeffer, C., Schowalter, J., & Shapiro, T. (1997). Evolution and revolution in child psychiatry: ADHD as a disorder of adaptation. *Journal of the American Academy of Child and Adolescent Psychiatry, 36*(12), 1672–1679; discussion 1679–1681.

Kabat-Zinn, J. (1982). An outpatient program in behavioral medicine for chronic pain patients based on the practice of mindfulness meditation: Theoretical considerations and preliminary results. *General Hospital Psychiatry, 4*(1), 33–47.

Kabat-Zinn, J. (1990). *Full catastrophe living: Using the wisdom of your body and mind to face stress, pain, and illness.* New York: Delacorte Press.

Kabat-Zinn, J., Lipworth, L., & Burney, R. (1985). The clinical use of mindfulness meditation for the self-regulation of chronic pain. *Journal of Behavioral Medicine, 8*(2), 163–190.

Kang, C., & Whittingham, K. (2010). Mindfulness: A dialogue between Buddhism and clinical psychology. *Mindfulness, 1*(3), 161–173.

Keith, J. R., Blackwood, M. E., Mathew, R. T., & Lecci, L. B. (2017). Self-reported mindful attention and awareness, go/no-go response-time variability, and attention-deficit hyperactivity disorder. *Mindfulness (NY), 8*(3), 765–774.

Kelly, K., & Ramundo, P. (2006). *You mean I'm not lazy, stupid or crazy?!: The classic self-help book for adults with attention deficit disorder.* New York: Scribner.

Kemper, K. J. (2017). Brief online mindfulness training: Immediate impact. *Journal of Evidence-Based Complementary and Alternative Medicine, 22*(1), 75–80.

Keng, S. L., Smoski, M. J., & Robins, C. J. (2011). Effects of mindfulness on psychological health: A review of empirical studies. *Clinical Psychology Review, 31*(6), 1041–1056.

Kessler, R. C., Adler, L., Barkley, R., Biederman, J., Conners, C. K., Demler, O., . . . Zaslavsky, A. M. (2006). The prevalence and correlates of adult ADHD in the United States: Results from the National Comorbidity Survey Replication. *American Journal of Psychiatry, 163*(4), 716–723.

Khoury, B., Lecomte, T., Fortin, G., Masse, M., Therien, P., Bouchard, V., . . . Hofmann, S. G. (2013). Mindfulness-based therapy: A comprehensive meta-analysis. *Clinical Psychology Review, 33*(6), 763–771.

Kiani, B., Hadianfard, H., & Mitchell, J. T. (2017). The impact of mindfulness meditation training on executive functions and emotion dysregulation in an Iranian sample of female adolescents with elevated attention-deficit/hyperactivity disorder symptoms. *Australian Journal of Psychology, 69*(4), 273–282.

Kichuk, S. A., Lebowitz, M. S., & Grover Adams, T. (2015). Can biomedical models of psychopathology interfere with cognitive-behavioral treatment processes? *The Behavior Therapist, 38*(7), 181–186.

Knouse, L. E., & Mitchell, J. T. (2015). Incautiously optimistic: Positively-valenced cognitive avoidance in Adult ADHD. *Cognitive and Behavioral Practice, 22*(2), 192–202.

Knouse, L. E., Mitchell, J. T., Kimbrel, N. A., & Anastopoulos, A. D. (2019). Development and evaluation of the ADHD Cognitions Scale for adults. *Journal of Attention Disorders, 23*(10), 1090–1100.

Knouse, L. E., Teller, J., & Brooks, M. A. (2017). Meta-analysis of cognitive-behavioral treatments for adult ADHD. *Journal of Consulting and Clinical Psychology, 85*(7), 737–750.

Knouse, L. E., Zvorsky, I., & Safren, S. A. (2013). Depression in adults with attention-deficit/hyperactivity disorder (ADHD): The mediating role of cognitive-behavioral factors. *Cognitive Therapy and Research, 37*(6), 1220–1232.

Kooj, J. J. S. (2013). *Adult ADHD: Diagnostic assessment and treatment* (3rd ed.). New York: Springer.

Krasner, M. S., Epstein, R. M., Beckman, H., Suchman, A. L., Chapman, B., Mooney, C. J., & Quill, T. E. (2009). Association of an educational program in mindful communication with burnout, empathy, and attitudes among primary care physicians. *Journal of the American Medical Association, 302*(12), 1284–1293.

Krcmar, K., & Horsman, T. (2016). *Mindfulness for study: From procrastination to action*. Aberdeen, Scotland: Inspired By Learning.

Krisanaprakornkit, T., Ngamjarus, C., Witoonchart, C., & Piyavhatkul, N. (2010). Meditation therapies for attention-deficit/hyperactivity disorder (ADHD). *Cochrane Database of Systematic Reviews*(6), CD006507.

Kurth, F., MacKenzie-Graham, A., Toga, A. W., & Luders, E. (2015). Shifting brain asymmetry: The link between meditation and structural lateralization. *Social Cognitive and Affective Neuroscience, 10*(1), 55–61.

Kuyken, W., Warren, F. C., Taylor, R. S., Whalley, B., Crane, C., Bondolfi, G., . . . Dalgleish, T. (2016). Efficacy of mindfulness-based cognitive therapy in prevention of depressive relapse: An individual patient data meta-analysis from randomized trials. *Journal of the American Medical Association Psychiatry, 73*(6), 565–574.

Kvaale, E. P., Haslam, N., & Gottdiener, W. H. (2013). The "side effects" of medicalization: A meta-analytic review of how biogenetic explanations affect stigma. *Clinical Psychology Review, 33*(6), 782–794.

Kwan, B. M., Dimidjian, S., & Rizvi, S. L. (2010). Treatment preference, engagement, and clinical improvement in pharmacotherapy versus psychotherapy for depression. *Behaviour Research and Therapy, 48*(8), 799–804.

Lebowitz, M. S., Pyun, J. J., & Ahn, W. K. (2014). Biological explanations of generalized anxiety disorder: Effects on beliefs about prognosis and responsibility. *Psychiatric Services, 65*(4), 498–503.

Lee, C. S. C., Ma, M. T., Ho, H. Y., Tsang, K. K., Zheng, Y. Y., & Wu, Z. Y. (2017). The effectiveness of mindfulness-based intervention in attention on individuals with ADHD: A systematic review. *Hong Kong Journal of Occupational Therapy, 30*(1), 33–41.

Levy, F., Hay, D. A., McStephen, M., Wood, C., & Waldman, I. (1997). Attention-deficit hyperactivity disorder: A category or a continuum?: Genetic analysis of a large-scale twin study. *Journal of the American Academy of Child and Adolescent Psychiatry, 36*(6), 737–744.

Liddle, E. B., Hollis, C., Batty, M. J., Groom, M. J., Totman, J. J., Liotti, M., . . . Liddle, P. F. (2011). Task-related default mode network modulation and inhibitory control in ADHD: Effects of motivation and methylphenidate. *Journal of Child Psychology and Psychiatry, 52*(7), 761–771.

Linehan, M. M. (1993). *Cognitive-behavioral treatment of borderline personality disorder*. New York: Guilford Press.

Loucks, E. B., Schuman-Olivier, Z., Britton, W. B., Fresco, D. M., Desbordes, G., Brewer, J. A., & Fulwiler, C. (2015). Mindfulness and cardiovascular disease risk: State of the evidence, plausible mechanisms, and theoretical framework. *Current Cardiology Reports, 17*(12), 112.

Lutz, A., Slagter, H. A., Dunne, J. D., & Davidson, R. J. (2008). Attention regulation and monitoring in meditation. *Trends in Cognitive Sciences, 12*(4), 163–169.

Lyzwinski, L. N., Caffery, L., Bambling, M., & Edirippulige, S. (2018). A systematic review of electronic mindfulness-based therapeutic interventions for weight, weight-related behaviors, and psychological stress. *Telemedicine Journal and E-Health, 24*(3), 173–184.

Martel, M. M. (2009). Research review: A new perspective on attention-deficit/hyperactivity disorder: Emotion dysregulation and trait models. *Journal of Child Psychology and Psychiatry, 50*(9), 1042–1051.

Mason, M. F., Norton, M. I., Van Horn, J. D., Wegner, D. M., Grafton, S. T., & Macrae, C. N. (2007). Wandering minds: The default network and stimulus-independent thought. *Science, 315*(5810), 393–395.

Matheson, L., Asherson, P., Wong, I. C., Hodgkins, P., Setyawan, J., Sasane, R., & Clifford, S. (2013). Adult ADHD patient experiences of impairment, service provision and clinical management in England: A qualitative study. *BMC Health Services Research, 13*, 184.

Menezes, C. B., & Bizarro, L. (2015). Effects of focused meditation on difficulties in emotion regulation and trait anxiety. *Psychology and Neuroscience, 8*(3), 350–365.

Menezes, C. B., de Paula Couto, M. C., Buratto, L. G., Erthal, F., Pereira, M. G., & Bizarro, L. (2013). The improvement of emotion and attention regulation after a 6-week training of focused meditation: A randomized controlled trial. *Evidence-Based Complementary and Alternative Medicine, 2013*, 984678.

Mennin, D. S., Heimberg, R. G., Turk, C. L., & Fresco, D. M. (2005). Preliminary evidence for an emotion dysregulation model of generalized anxiety disorder. *Behaviour Research and Therapy, 43*(10), 1281–1310.

Merzenich, M. M., Nahum, M., & Van Vleet, T. M. (2013). Neuroplasticity: Introduction. *Progress in Brain Research, 207*, xxi–xxvi.

Merzenich, M. M., Van Vleet, T. M., & Nahum, M. (2014). Brain plasticity-based therapeutics. *Frontiers in Human Neuroscience, 8*, 385.

Mikolasek, M., Berg, J., Witt, C. M., & Barth, J. (2018). Effectiveness of mindfulness- and relaxation-based ehealth interventions for patients with medical conditions: A systematic review and synthesis. *International Journal of Behavioral Medicine, 25*(1), 1–16.

Mitchell, J. T., Bates, A., & Zylowska, L. (2018). Adverse events in mindfulness-based interventions for ADHD. *The ADHD Report, 26*(2), 15–18.

Mitchell, J. T., Benson, J. W., Knouse, L. K., Kimbrel, N. A., & Anastopolous, A. D. (2013). Are negative automatic thoughts associated with ADHD in adulthood? *Cognitive Therapy and Research, 37*(4), 851–859.

Mitchell, J. T., McIntyre, E. M., English, J. S., Dennis, M. F., Beckham, J. C., & Kollins, S. H. (2017). A pilot trial of mindfulness meditation training for ADHD in adulthood: Impact on core symptoms, executive functioning, and emotion dysregulation. *Journal of Attention Disorders, 21*(13), 1105–1120.

Mitchell, J. T., Robertson, C. D., Anastopolous, A. D., Nelson-Gray, R. O., & Kollins, S. H. (2012). Emotion dysregulation and emotional impulsivity among adults diagnosed with attention-deficit/hyperactivity disorder: Results of a preliminary study. *Journal of Psychopathology and Behavioral Assessment, 34*(4), 510–519.

Mitchell, J. T., Zylowska, L., & Kollins, S. H. (2015). Mindfulness meditation training for attention-deficit/hyperactivity disorder in adulthood: Current empirical support, treatment overview, and future directions. *Cognitive and Behavioral Practice, 22*(2), 172–191.

Modesto-Lowe, V., Farahmand, P., Chaplin, M., & Sarro, L. (2015). Does mindfulness meditation improve attention in attention deficit hyperactivity disorder? *World Journal of Psychiatry, 5*(4), 397–403.

Mowlem, F. D., Skirrow, C., Reid, P., Maltezos, S., Nijjar, S. K., Merwood, A., . . . Asherson, P. (2019). Validation of the mind excessively wandering scale and the relationship of mind wandering to impairment in adult ADHD. *Journal of Attention Disorders, 23*(6), 624–634. [Epub ahead of print]

Moyer, C. A., Donnelly, M. P., Anderson, J. C., Valek, K. C., Huckaby, S. J., Wiederholt, D. A., . . . Rice, B. L. (2011). Frontal electroencephalographic asymmetry associated with positive emotion is produced by very brief meditation training. *Psychological Science, 22*(10), 1277–1279.

Mrazek, M. D., Franklin, M. S., Phillips, D. T., Baird, B., & Schooler, J. W. (2013). Mindfulness training improves working memory capacity and GRE performance while reducing mind wandering. *Psychological Science, 24*(5), 776–781.

Mrazek, M. D., Smallwood, J., & Schooler, J. W. (2012). Mindfulness and mind-wandering: Finding convergence through opposing constructs. *Emotion, 12*(3), 442–448.

Mukerji Househam, A., & Solanto, M. V. (2016). Mindfulness as an intervention for ADHD. *The ADHD Report, 24*(2), 1–13.

Nigg, J. T. (2006). *What causes ADHD?: Understanding what goes wrong and why*. New York: Guilford Press.

Noordali, F., Cumming, J., & Thompson, J. L. (2017). Effectiveness of mindfulness-based interventions on physiological and psychological complications in adults with diabetes: A systematic review. *Journal of Health Psychology, 22*(8), 965–983.

Ogrodniczuk, J. S., Joyce, A. S., & Piper, W. E. (2005). Strategies for reducing patient-initiated premature termination of psychotherapy. *Harvard Review of Psychiatry, 13*(2), 57–70.

Oikonomou, M. T., Arvanitis, M., & Sokolove, R. L. (2017). Mindfulness training for smoking cessation: A meta-analysis of randomized-controlled trials. *Journal of Health Psychology, 22*(14), 1841–1850.

Orlov, M., & Kohlenberger, N. (2014). *The couple's guide to thriving with ADHD*. Plantation, FL: Specialty Press.

Passarotti, A. M., Sweeney, J. A., & Pavuluri, M. N. (2010). Emotion processing influences working memory circuits in pediatric bipolar disorder and attention-deficit/hyperactivity disorder. *Journal of the American Academy of Child and Adolescent Psychiatry, 49*(10), 1064–1080.

Pera, G., & Robin, A. L. (Eds.). (2016). *Adult ADHD-focused couple therapy: Clinical interventions*. New York: Routledge.

Peterson, B. S., Potenza, M. N., Wang, Z., Zhu, H., Martin, A., Marsh, R., . . . Yu, S. (2009). An FMRI study of the effects of psychostimulants on default-mode processing during Stroop task performance in youths with ADHD. *American Journal of Psychiatry, 166*(11), 1286–1294.

Philipsen, A., Richter, H., Peters, J., Alm, B., Sobanski, E., Colla, M., . . . Hesslinger, B. (2007). Structured group psychotherapy in adults with attention deficit hyperactivity disorder: Results of an open multicentre study. *Journal of Nervous and Mental Disease, 195*(12), 1013–1019.

Piet, J., Wurtzen, H., & Zachariae, R. (2012). The effect of mindfulness-based therapy on symptoms of anxiety and depression in adult cancer patients and survivors: A systematic review and meta-analysis. *Journal of Consulting and Clinical Psychology, 80*(6), 1007–1020.

Poissant, H., Mendrek, A., Talbot, N., Khoury, B., & Nolan, J. (2019). Behavioral and cognitive impacts of mindfulness-based interventions on adults with attention deficit hyperactivity disorder: A systematic review. *Behavioural Neurology, 2019* Article ID 5682050.

Posner, M. I., Sheese, B. E., Odludas, Y., & Tang, Y. (2006). Analyzing and shaping human attentional networks. *Neural Networks, 19*(9), 1422–1429.

Pozuelos, J. P., Mead, B. R., Rueda, M. R., & Malinowski, P. (2019). Short-term mindful breath awareness training improves inhibitory control and response monitoring. *Progress in Brain Research, 244*, 137–163.

Raes, F., Pommier, E., Neff, K. D., & Van Gucht, D. (2011). Construction and factorial validation of a short form of the Self-Compassion Scale. *Clinical Psychology and Psychotherapy, 18*(3), 250–255.

Raichle, M. E., MacLeod, A. M., Snyder, A. Z., Powers, W. J., Gusnard, D. A., & Shulman, G. L. (2001). A default mode of brain function. *Proceeding of the National Academy of Sciences of the USA, 98*(2), 676–682.

Ramsay, J. R. (2017). Assessment and monitoring of treatment response in adult ADHD patients: Current perspectives. *Neuropsychiatric Disease and Treatment, 13*, 221–232.

Ramsay, J. R. (2020). *Rethinking adult ADHD: Helping clients turn intentions into actions*. Washington, DC: American Psychological Association.

Renshaw, T. L., & Cook, C. R. (2017). Introduction to the Special Issue: Mindfulness in the schools—Historical roots, current status, and future directions. *Psychology in the Schools, 54*(1), 5–12.

Rosenberg, M. B. (1999). *Non-violent communication: A language of compassion*. Encinitas, CA: PuddleDancer Press.

Roth, R. M., Isquith P. K., & Gioia, G. A. (2005). *Behavior Rating Inventory of Executive Function–Adult Version (BRIEF-A)*. Lutz, FL: Psychological Assessment Resources.

Roth, R. M., Lance, C. E., Isquith, P. K., Fischer, A. S., & Giancola, P. R. (2013). Confirmatory factor analysis of the Behavior Rating Inventory of Executive Function—adult version in healthy adults and application to attention-deficit/hyperactivity disorder. *Archives of Clinical Neuropsychology, 28*(5), 425–434.

Rubia, K., Alegria, A., & Brinson, H. (2014). Imaging the ADHD brain: Disorder-specificity, medication effects and clinical translation. *Expert Review of Neurotherapeutics, 14*(5), 519–538.

Safren, S. A., Perlman, C. A., Sprich, S., & Otto, M. W. (2005). *Mastering your adult ADHD: A cognitive-behavioral treatment program therapist guide.* New York: Oxford University Press.

Safren, S. A., Sprich, S. E., Cooper-Vince, C., Knouse, L. E., & Lerner, J. A. (2010). Life impairments in adults with medication-treated ADHD. *Journal of Attention Disorders, 13*(5), 524–531.

Safren, S. A., Sprich, S., Mimiaga, M. J., Surman, C., Knouse, L., Groves, M., & Otto, M. W. (2010). Cognitive behavioral therapy vs relaxation with educational support for medication-treated adults with ADHD and persistent symptoms: A randomized controlled trial. *Journal of the American Medical Association, 304*(8), 875–880.

Schmidt, A. T. (2016). The ethics and politics of mindfulness-based interventions. *Journal of Medical Ethics, 42*(7), 450–454.

Schoenberg, P. L., Hepark, S., Kan, C. C., Barendregt, H. P., Buitelaar, J. K., & Speckens, A. E. (2014). Effects of mindfulness-based cognitive therapy on neurophysiological correlates of performance monitoring in adult attention-deficit/hyperactivity disorder. *Clinical Neurophysiology, 125*(7), 1407–1416.

Searight, H. R., Robertson, K., Smith, T., Perkins, S., & Searight, B. K. (2012). Complementary and alternative therapies for pediatric attention deficit hyperactivity disorder: A descriptive review. *International Scholarly Research Network Psychiatry, 2012,* 804127.

Segal, Z. V., Williams, J. M. G., & Teasdale, J. D. (2002). *Mindfulness-based cognitive therapy for depression: A new approach to preventing relapse.* New York: Guilford Press.

Shaw, P., Stringaris, A., Nigg, J., & Leibenluft, E. (2014). Emotion dysregulation in attention deficit hyperactivity disorder. *American Journal of Psychiatry, 171*(3), 276–293.

Sibley, M. H., Mitchell, J. T., & Becker, S. P. (2016). Method of adult diagnosis influences estimated persistence of childhood ADHD: A systematic review of longitudinal studies. *Lancet Psychiatry, 3*(12), 1157–1165.

Sibley, M. H., Pelham, W. E., Molina, B. S., Gnagy, E. M., Waxmonsky, J. G., Waschbusch, D. A., . . . Kuriyan, A. B. (2012). When diagnosing ADHD in young adults emphasize informant reports, DSM items, and impairment. *Journal of Consulting and Clinical Psychology, 80*(6), 1052–1061.

Siebelink, N. M., Asherson, P., Antonova, E., Bogels, S. M., Speckens, A. E., Buitelaar, J. K., & Greven, C. U. (2019). Genetic and environmental aetiologies of associations between dispositional mindfulness and ADHD traits: A population-based twin study. *European Child and Adolescent Psychiatry, 28*(9), 1241–1251.

Smalley, S. L., Loo, S. K., Hale, T. S., Shrestha, A., McGough, J., Flook, L., & Reise, S. (2009). Mindfulness and attention deficit hyperactivity disorder. *Journal of Clinical Psychology, 65*(10), 1087–1098.

Smallwood, J., & Schooler, J. W. (2006). The restless mind. *Psychological Bulletin, 132*(6), 946–958.

Solanto, M. V., Marks, D. J., Wasserstein, J., Mitchell, K., Abikoff, H., Alvir, J. M., & Kofman, M. D. (2010). Efficacy of meta-cognitive therapy for adult ADHD. *American Journal of Psychiatry, 167*(8), 958–968.

Sonuga-Barke, E. J., & Castellanos, F. X. (2007). Spontaneous attentional fluctuations in impaired states and pathological conditions: A neurobiological hypothesis. *Neuroscience and Biobehavioral Reviews, 31*(7), 977–986.

Spencer, T., Biederman, J., Wilens, T. E., & Faraone, S. V. (1998). Adults with attention-deficit/hyperactivity disorder: A controversial diagnosis. *Journal of Clinical Psychiatry, 59*(Suppl. 7), 59–68.

Strayhorn, J. M., Jr. (2002). Self-control: Toward systematic training programs. *Journal of the American Academy of Child and Adolescent Psychiatry, 41*(1), 17–27.

Strohmeier, C. W., Rosenfield, B., DiTomasso, R. A., & Ramsay, J. R. (2016). Assessment of the relationship between self-reported cognitive distortions and adult ADHD, anxiety, depression, and hopelessness. *Psychiatry Research, 238*, 153–158.

Swift, J. K., & Greenberg, R. P. (2012). Premature discontinuation in adult psychotherapy: A meta-analysis. *Journal of Consulting and Clinical Psychology, 80*(4), 547–559.

Swift, K. D., Hall, C. L., Marimuttu, V., Redstone, L., Sayal, K., & Hollis, C. (2013). Transition to adult mental health services for young people with attention deficit/hyperactivity disorder (ADHD): A qualitative analysis of their experiences. *BMC Psychiatry, 13*, 74.

Tang, Y. Y., Ma, Y., Wang, J., Fan, Y., Feng, S., Lu, Q., . . . Posner, M. I. (2007). Short-term meditation training improves attention and self-regulation. *Proceedings of the National Academy of Sciences of the USA, 104*(43), 17152–17156.

Tang, Y. Y., & Posner, M. I. (2013). Special issue on mindfulness neuroscience. *Social Cognitive and Affective Neuroscience, 8*(1), 1–3.

Taylor, V. A., Daneault, V., Grant, J., Scavone, G., Breton, E., Roffe-Vidal, S., . . . Beauregard, M. (2013). Impact of meditation training on the default mode network during a restful state. *Social Cognitive and Affective Neuroscience, 8*(1), 4–14.

Teper, R., Segal, Z. V., & Inzlicht, M. (2013). Inside the mindful mind: How mindfulness enhances emotion regulation through improvements in executive control. *Current Directions in Psychological Science, 22*(6), 449–454.

Thomas, A., & Chess, S. (1977). *Temperament and development*. New York: Brunner/Mazel.

Thupten, J. (2018). The question of mindfulness' connection with ethics and compassion. *Current Opinion in Psychology, 28*, 71–75.

Uliando, A. (2010). *Mindfulness training for the management of children with ADHD*. Geelong, Australia: School of Psychology, Deakin University.

Van Dam, N. T., van Vugt, M. K., Vago, D. R., Schmalzl, L., Saron, C. D., Olendzki, A., . . . Meyer, D. E. (2018). Mind the hype: A critical evaluation and prescriptive agenda for research on mindfulness and meditation. *Perspectives on Psychological Science, 13*(1), 36–61.

van de Weijer-Bergsma, E., Formsma, A. R., de Bruin, E. I., & Bögels, S. M. (2012). The effectiveness of mindfulness training on behavioral problems and attentional functioning in adolescents with ADHD. *Journal of Child and Family Studies, 21*(5), 775–787.

van der Oord, S., Bögels, S. M., & Peijnenburg, D. (2012). The effectiveness of mindfulness training for children with ADHD and mindful parenting for their parents. *Journal of Child and Family Studies, 21*(1), 139–147.

Vidal, R., Bosch, R., Nogueira, M., Gomez-Barros, N., Valero, S., Palomar, G., . . . Ramos-Quiroga, J. A. (2013). Psychoeducation for adults with attention deficit hyperactivity disorder vs. cognitive behavioral group therapy: A randomized controlled pilot study. *Journal of Nervous and Mental Disease, 201*(10), 894–900.

White, H. A., & Shah, P. (2011). Creative style and achievement in adults with attention-deficit/hyperactivity disorder. *Personality and Individual Differences, 50*(5), 673–677.

Wilens, T. E., Biederman, J., & Spencer, T. J. (1998). Pharmacotherapy of attention deficit hyperactivity disorder in adults. *CNS Drugs, 9*(5), 347–356.

Wilens, T. E., Spencer, T. J., & Biederman, J. (2002). A review of the pharmacotherapy of adults with attention-deficit/hyperactivity disorder. *Journal of Attention Disorders, 5*(4), 189–202.

Willcutt, E. G. (2012). The prevalence of DSM-IV attention-deficit/hyperactivity disorder: A meta-analytic review. *Neurotherapeutics, 9*(3), 490–499.

Wolkin, J. R. (2015). Cultivating multiple aspects of attention through mindfulness meditation accounts for psychological well-being through decreased rumination. *Psychology Research and Behavioral Management, 8*, 171–180.

Wymbs, B. T., & Molina, B. S. G. (2015). Integrative couples group treatment for emerging adults with ADHD symptoms. *Cognitive and Behavioral Practice, 22*(2), 161–171.

Xue, J., Zhang, Y., & Huang, Y. (2019). A meta-analytic investigation of the impact of mindfulness-based interventions on ADHD symptoms. *Medicine (Baltimore), 98*(23), e15957.

Young, Z., Moghaddam, N., & Tickle, A. (2020). The efficacy of cognitive behavioral therapy for adults with ADHD: A systematic review and meta-analysis of randomized controlled trials. *Journal of Attention Disorders, 24*(6), 875–888. [Epub ahead of print]

Zainal, N. Z., Booth, S., & Huppert, F. A. (2013). The efficacy of mindfulness-based stress reduction on mental health of breast cancer patients: A meta-analysis. *Psychooncology, 22*(7), 1457–1465.

Zeidan, F., Johnson, S. K., Diamond, B. J., David, Z., & Goolkasian, P. (2010). Mindfulness meditation improves cognition: Evidence of brief mental training. *Consciousness and Cognition, 19*(2), 597–605.

Zgierska, A., Rabago, D., Chawla, N., Kushner, K., Koehler, R., & Marlatt, A. (2009). Mindfulness meditation for substance use disorders: A systematic review. *Substance Abuse, 30*(4), 266–294.

Zhang, J., Diaz-Roman, A., & Cortese, S. (2018). Meditation-based therapies for attention-deficit/hyperactivity disorder in children, adolescents and adults: A systematic review and meta-analysis. *Evidence-Based Mental Health, 21*(3), 87–94.

Zylowska, L. (2012). *The Mindfulness Prescription for Adult ADHD: An 8-step program for strengthening attention, managing emotions, and achieving goals*. Boston: Trumpeter Books.

Zylowska, L., Ackerman, D. L., Yang, M. H., Futrell, J. L., Horton, N. L., Hale, T. S., . . . Smalley, S. L. (2008). Mindfulness meditation training in adults and adolescents with ADHD: A feasibility study. *Journal of Attention Disorders, 11*(6), 737–746.

Zylowska, L., Smalley, S. L., & Schwartz, J. M. (2009). Mindful awareness and ADHD. In F. Didonna (Ed.), *Clinical handbook of mindfulness* (pp. 319–338). New York: Springer.

Index

Note. *f* or *t* following a page number indicates a figure or a table.

E

F

G

H

N

O

P

R

S

T

V

W

Y